Living with Environmental Illness

Stephen B. Edelson, MD
with Jan Statman

TAYLOR PUBLISHING COMPANY, DALLAS, TEXAS

Published by Taylor Publishing Company
1550 West Mockingbird Lane
Dallas, Texas 75235

Book design by Mark McGarry
Set in Goudy and Goudy Sans

Library of Congress Cataloging-in-Publication Data
Living with environmental illness / Stephen Edelson, with Jan Statman.
p.   cm.   Includes index.
ISBN 087833-968-x
1. Multiple chemical sensitivity. I. Statman, Jan Berliner. II. Title
RB152.6.E34   1998
615.9'02—DC21   98–9364
CIP

Printed in the United States of America
10 9 8 7 6 5 4 3 2 1

To Carol, whose love and support has been my greatest asset.
To Richard and Dana for their unyeilding love and support.
To Alex, Bradley, and Joshua, who make life worth living.

STEPHEN B. EDELSON, M.D.

To Max, who hung the moon, and to Charles Barry,
Louis Craig, and Sherry Michelle, who bring
sparkle to the stars.

JAN STATMAN

Contents

Ask the Doctor

IN THIS CHAPTER, Dr. Edelson answers the ten most commonly asked questions about multiple chemical sensitivity.

1. *What is the difference between allergy and sensitivity?*
   They have no relationship. Allergy is an alteration in reactivity that is acquired and initiated by exposure to a specific allergen in the environment. Multiple chemical sensitivity is a disease process in which an individual reacts in a negative way to levels of chemicals in the environment that are below the levels that would be considered a problem for the average individual.

2. *Do people ever get cured of multiple chemical sensitivity?*
   Cure isn't a really good word when you are dealing with individual environmental and genetically related problems. You can control the illness, but I don't believe you can cure it. With the appropriate care you can probably improve your

well-being between 85 and 95 percent. People can certainly be made comfortable if they are careful.

3. *What's the best way for people with multiple chemical sensitivity to cope with their illness?*

    Follow the advice of a physician who is highly skilled in all aspects of environmental and nutritional medicine. He or she will work with you to control your illness so that you may lead a reasonably normal life.

4. *Does it matter where a person who has multiple chemical sensitivity lives?*

    Absolutely! The best place for you to live is at the beach or in the mountains—as far away from any farming or industry as possible.

5. *Is multiple chemical sensitivity contagious?*

    No. You can't catch it from another person. You can only get it from environmental toxic injury and usually only if you are genetically predisposed, which is something we can't measure.

6. *What causes multiple chemical sensitivity?*

    A reaction to toxic chemicals in the air, water, and food is the cause. The nature of this reaction is to some degree dependent on the tissue involved; the pharmacological nature of the substance involved; the duration, concentration, and virulence of the exposure; indirect susceptibility, both nutritional and genetic; and total toxic load at the time of exposure.

7. *Is multiple chemical sensitivity genetic in origin?*

    If you mean can you inherit it like curly hair or blue eyes, I would have to say no. However, some people seem to have genetic predispositions, similar to a predisposition to alcoholism, to developing multiple chemical sensitivity.

8. *When does multiple chemical sensitivity occur?*

Multiple chemical sensitivity can occur rapidly after a massive chemical exposure. It can also occur slowly, as the result of cumulative low-level exposures over a period of time. It often follows exposures to low levels of chemicals following some kind of traumatic event such as childbirth, influenza immunization, major surgery, or an injury.

9. *What are the major symptoms of multiple chemical sensitivity?*

Everyone has different symptoms, but the symptoms usually include headaches, respiratory problems, sneezing, runny nose, irritated eyes, nasal problems, neurocognitive difficulties, memory disorder, dizziness, muscle pain and weakness, numbness, joint pain, depression, disorientation, visual disturbances, heart irregularities, unexplained skin rashes, and extreme, unrelenting fatigue.

10. *Is multiple chemical sensitivity life threatening?*

Only if nothing is done about the cause of multiple chemical sensitivity and if a person continues to be exposed to toxic materials. If the damage is left untreated, it can result in damage to organs and eventually death.

What Is Multiple Chemical Sensitivity?

IN SPITE OF what you may have heard, all chemicals are not necessarily bad for you. In fact, chemicals are the building blocks of life on planet earth. It is only when the human body is assaulted by an irresponsible barrage of toxic chemicals that have been spewed into our environment that we start to get into trouble.

Multiple chemical sensitivity is an environmental illness in which the environment itself makes people sick. It is an adverse reaction to toxic chemicals in our air, water, food, drugs, and surroundings even when they are at levels below those that are officially considered to be harmful to the general public.

This acquired disorder can affect many of the body's different organs and systems. In some people it can result from a single severe reaction to a single chemical, while in other people it can be the cumulative effect of low-level exposures to one or a variety of chemicals that take place over a long period of time. It is brought about by a number of factors, including the timing of the first exposure, and is affected by the person's biochemical individuality. To make matters even more complicated, it can affect any number of the body's biological mechanisms and systems. The appearance of harmful reactions depends on the tissues or organs involved; the pharmacological nature of the toxin; the susceptibility of the person who is affected, including his or her genetic make-up and nutritional state; the length of time of the exposure; and the total load of chemical exposures endured over the time of exposure.

For environmentally sensitive people, chronic exposure, even at low levels, can mark the start of multiple chemical sensitivity. Once it has been triggered, a chain of events can damage both immune mechanisms and nonimmune systems. Toxicity can result in end-organ disease, such as specific illnesses, disability, and even death.

Chronic cumulative low-level exposure may result in immune system problems; brain damage; liver, kidney, and heart conditions; neurological disorders; autoimmunity; birth defects; and any number of other diseases and malfunctions. However, low-level chemical exposure is thought to cause an assortment of damages so minor that the body doesn't recognize it's in danger until the injuries have reached a critical point. The body often does not even start responding to these chemical assaults until after irreversible damage has been done.

Surprisingly, environmental illness is not a new idea. Elements in the environment have always made people sick. Archaeological evidence indicates that the earliest people developed illnesses from inhaling the smoke of their cooking fires. They were forced to invent ways to vent the smoke from their primitive dwellings. Ancient metallurgy put toxic waste into water systems. The lead that was used in water pipes and in cooking pottery is generally considered to have contributed to the fall of the Roman Empire, because many members of the upper classes experienced mental and physical problems as a direct result of lead poisoning.

But it wasn't until the Industrial Revolution that humankind managed to substantially increase the rate of new afflictions. When Lewis Carroll's Alice met The Mad Hatter she recognized that he was remarkably loony, but these days few of us attribute his bizarre behavior to the occupational hazards of Victorian hatmakers. Everybody in Lewis Carroll's time knew that the constant exposure to mercury compounds used in making felt caused hatmakers to suffer from debilitating mental illnesses and early death.

Silk workers in the Paterson, New Jersey, silk mills rioted early in the twentieth century, largely in protest against the introduction of fibers containing synthetic dyes, which they believed were causing them and their families to suffer from an unusually high incidence of cancer and neurological diseases.

Coal miners have always been subject to a host of horrifying dangers, but one of the most terrifying threats they faced was an accumulation of deadly mine gas. To combat sudden death, a canary in a cage became an early example of poison detection. It was not unusual to see powerful coal miners marching off to work carrying a little canary, singing merrily away inside its cage. Although the canary often became the miner's constant companion, it was not a pet. It was a potential life saver.

The miners were aware that a canary was more quickly susceptible to poison gases than a human. If the canary died, the miners knew it was time to flee the mine. In another use, a canary in a cage was lowered into a new or suspicious mine shaft before the men went down. If the canary survived, work would progress, but if the canary was brought up dead, the miners knew the shaft was poisoned.

Our increasingly polluted environment has made the whole world as dangerous as those mine shafts. Chemically sensitive people are not unlike the canaries in the coal mines. Their sickness warns us of what we all may face if we cannot or will not take steps to restore our environment.

We are the first generation of our species to be exposed to this massive overload of chemicals. With the human system under attack as it has never been before, our bodies are developing new and more debilitating illnesses to add to the list of old, familiar miseries. Since hazardous chemicals can be all around us, we need to take personal responsibility to make educated choices and learn what can be done to protect ourselves.

Increasing numbers of people are suffering from multiple chemical sensitivity. As far back as 1987, the National Research Council's Board of Environmental Studies and Toxicology published "Health Risks from Exposure to Common Indoor Household Products in Allergic or Chemically Diseased Persons" (July 1, 1987) in which it estimated that 15 to 30 percent of the population may be sensitive to chemicals in their surroundings whether they are at work or at home.

Since that time, multiple chemical sensitivity has been on the rise. Although the precise number of people suffering from multiple chemical sensitivity is not known, this disease is real. It exists and can be linked to concrete biological causes. Even though a single, specific test has not yet been developed to diagnose this illness, and even though its exact mechanisms remain unclear, the symptoms are disabling more and more productive members of society.

The increase may be related to the rise in the production of synthetic organic chemicals as well as to the construction of tighter and increasingly insulated schools, homes, and office buildings, which has resulted in indoor and outdoor air pollution.

There are several theories on how these exposures are poisoning people. The one recurring idea is that chemical sensitivity may not be primarily immune system dysfunction. It is probably central nervous system damage with secondary endocrine and immune system involvement and is characterized by damage throughout the body.

This painful, frustrating, mysterious, often baffling disease has also been called the "twentieth-century allergy," "total allergy syndrome," and "twentieth-century disease." Those who find themselves suffering from it come up against such confusing terms as *biological individuality*, *adaptation* or *masking*, *spreading*, and the *switch phenomenon*.

Biochemical Individuality

With all the chemicals surrounding us, it is easy to wonder why everyone in the world is not suffering from this disease. Fortunately, we are all biochemically different, and we all deal with external environments in a unique way. Some of us are more seriously at risk from exposures at work or at home. Others are able to withstand more exposure without suffering the worst effects.

Although we are seldom aware of it when it is happening, every chemical we come in contact with makes its way into our bodies one way or another. Sometimes these chemicals remain in our bodies for years. Whether the intrusion comes through air, water, food, or physical contact, each of us responds differently.

It isn't difficult to understand the way biochemical individuality affects our response to sickness. Suppose you attend a holiday party with a friend. It is midwinter and you are confined to a small room in which the other guests are coughing and sniffling. Within days you are also coughing and sniffling. You have come down with a terrible cold, but the friend who attended the party with you is just fine. You were both subjected to the cold virus at the same time, in the same place, and under the same circumstances, but you both responded differently to the virus. At that particular moment, your friend was in a position to fight that particular virus and to conquer it. You were not.

Suppose you work in an office or business where the chemical odors are so strong they give your coworkers a headache, although you barely notice there is a problem. Here again, biochemical individuality has allowed you to responded differently to the chemical affront.

Since everyone is equipped to handle pollutants in a unique way, biochemical individuality contributes to how intensely you may react to toxic exposures and how susceptible you will be to developing chemical sensitivity. Your potential susceptibility depends on many things, including genetic make up, total toxic body load, nutritional state at the time of exposure, and even the nutritional health and toxic body burden during your mother's pregnancy. More than that, we have differing quantities and interactions of carbohydrates, fats, proteins, enzymes, vitamins, minerals, and enzyme detoxication parameters that respond to environmental factors and determine the ability to process all the substances we encounter. Most people don't experience chemical sensitivity because they have strong detoxication systems. If your liver, kidneys, or gastrointestinal tract function normally, there is a good chance you will not suffer from the buildup of certain chemicals. Biochemical individuality allows some of us to clear the body of individual noxious substances, while others collect them.

Total Body Load

The total body load includes all the chemicals and metals the body has absorbed or stored, as well as all those problems to which the body must respond or adapt. These may be chemical or they may be biological, such as molds, pollens, bacteria, or viruses. They may be physical, such as cold, heat, or radiation. Or they may even be psychological or the result of past experiences and chemical offenses.

These physical factors are combined with the toxic chemicals we take in, such things as pesticides, formaldehydes, phenols, and the components of car exhausts. These are compounded by the total loads of things like lead, ozone, cadmium, cyanide, chlorine, heavy metals, and nitrous oxides. Add to this burden the load imposed by such biological factors as molds, bacteria, protozoa, dusts, amoebae, pollens, worms, viruses, parasites, and even the quality of the food you eat. Then consider psychological or emotional factors that significantly affect your ability to cope with those things and make it difficult to maintain stability in the face of acute and chronic exposures. This is your total body load.

It is necessary to remember that the total body load is not fixed. It can be increased by stress, infection, lack of sleep, lack of exercise, or specific exposure to various chemical substances that may be experienced over a period of time. The total body load is subjected to the biochemical individuality of the specific person and how much that person's body can tolerate. It is reasonable to believe that chemically sensitive people may be more susceptible to the effects of chemical compounds than the rest of us.

How does the body become overloaded? When we pack for a trip, most of us fill our suitcases full of the clothing and toiletry articles we are going to need while we are away. We manage to stuff everything we possibly can stuff into that suitcase until it is so full we have to sit on it to make it close, straining the fasteners to hold the burden of our personal items. When the suitcase becomes so full that we can't put any more in it, we are in danger of watching it burst at the seams. Imagine the body as this stuffed suitcase. If we limit the number of pollutants we put into it, we're in good shape; but if we continue to stuff more and more into it, we are in danger of overloading it.

The body must cope with the total load of pollutants we take in from everything we eat, drink, touch, inhale, or absorb through our skin. These must be used, expelled, or compartmentalized. When the body becomes overloaded, it will develop multiple chemical sensitivity with its confusing array of adaptation, bipolarity, spreading, and switching.

Multiple chemical sensitivity is developed as a two-stage process. There is an induction and then triggering. The specific exposures that cause a person to become sick with multiple chemical sensitivity and then trigger symptoms will vary from person to person.

Induction

The first stage of multiple chemical sensitivity involves either a high-level exposure or continuous low-level exposures to various substances, or a combination of high- and low-level exposures. Low-level exposures may be compounded after a period of time. One person will develop multiple chemical sensitivity after one acute exposure to certain pesticides, to certain solvents, or to formaldehyde. Another person will develop multiple chemical sensitivity only after weeks, months or even years of low-level exposures to pesticides, cleaning solutions, or gases released as the result of remodeling activities.

Triggering

Once the disease has begun, the second stage of multiple chemical sensitivity involves exposures to other substances that will trigger symptoms. Triggering can be brought on by exposure to the same chemical or chemicals that started the illness or by exposure to different chemicals altogether. It can be brought on by much lower levels of chemicals than those that initially started the illness.

Some examples of triggers that cause a recurrence of symptoms in a great many people include tobacco smoke, perfumes, pesticides, office copiers, printed books, glues, newspapers, and leather. Indoor air pollution exposures are responsible for the greatest numbers of multiple chemical sensitivity illness clusters. In some instances sick building syndrome may be a precursor to multiple chemical sensitivity.

Masking

One of the factors that complicates the process of unraveling chemical poisoning is masking, or adaptation. People who are gradually exposed to some form of chemical as a continuing part of their lives become adapted to it. People are capable of adapting to all sorts of harmful things in order to continue living their lives as normally as possible.

A simplistic explanation of the extremely complicated process of masking is that some people form a sensitivity to a particular chemical, but their bodies cover up the unpleasant symptoms. Instead of feeling sick when they are exposed to the chemical, they actually form an addiction to it. If an affected person doesn't get a regular dose of that chemical, the body will go into withdrawal much like the withdrawal associated with drug or alcohol addiction. But while obvious symptoms are being controlled by the masking process, the body's internal damage continues to progress unchecked.

Every woman will recognize the experience of trying a new perfume. It will have a delightful scent at first, but after a few moments, certainly after a few hours, she will no longer be able to smell the perfume she is wearing even though other people may remark about how lovely it is. Her body has masked the scent. Such masking can have serious consequences. Victor's story can clearly explain this.

Victor is a taxi driver who works on the city streets, driving his taxi all day long. Although the fumes and auto emissions bothered him when he first took his job, he has become so accustomed to driving on the city's streets he no longer notices them. But even though his body has adapted, the fumes are still damaging to him.

In addition, it is interesting to know that Victor chooses to spend most of his holidays taking long driving trips, and he spends his days off hanging out at the garage to visit with his coworkers. The sad fact is that he's become addicted to the same auto fumes that are making him sick. He doesn't know it, but he's not really hanging out at the garage to enjoy the good companionship of his coworkers. He's there to smell the fumes!

All smokers will remember the first time they inhaled a cigarette behind the barn. Their eyes burned, they choked and coughed, their throats were irritated, and they may have become nauseated. It was a totally unpleasant experience. But with time, and with continued smoking, smokers adapt to the unpleasant effects and experience only the pleasurable sensations of nicotine reaching the brain. When they attempt to stop smoking, they will suffer withdrawal symptoms. They will have headaches, be exhausted, drowsy, hot, cold, irritable, and moody, possibly even experiencing difficulty concentrating or extreme weight gain.

After they have successfully kicked the habit, they may find that being in a smoke-filled room causes them to suffer painful discomfort. You will often hear reformed smokers proclaiming long and loud about the disgusting effects of that harmful habit. They are not necessarily being self-righteous in the company of smokers. The presence of smoke makes them seriously uncomfortable. They have become deadapted, so the original unpleasant sensations have returned and they are able to experience normal reactions to the irritants. Avoiding exposure to the masked chemicals causes the warning signals to reappear, often more intensely than before.

The insidious difference between substance addictions and a masking addiction to chemicals is that in masking addiction to chemicals, a person will have no idea such addiction is taking place. After all, you know what you're doing when you're smoking or drinking. You can't always know what's happening to you when you are involuntarily subjected to harmful chemicals.

Adaptation is a survival mechanism that unfortunately also makes warning signals disappear. A person adapts to constant toxic exposure in order to survive but, at the same time, suffers a long-term decrease in efficient functioning and perhaps longevity. Because of adaptation or tolerance, the patient's total body load may increase undetected because the perception of a cause-and-effect relationship has been lost.

With no warning symptoms, repeated exposures may continue and cause damage to the immune and enzyme detoxification systems. The eventual result of continued toxic exposure over a period of days, weeks, months, and years is organ failure.

Bipolarity

There is no question that masking causes problems. Those people who are in an adapted state often misinterpret their experience as being normal. After first exposure, or even after occasional exposures, the body may be stimulated by the offending substance, creating an energized "high." Continued exposures will wear down the body's defenses and cause the stimulatory phase to recede. A down period will then set in.

At this time, symptoms of disabling depression and exhaustion develop. The frequency of these ups and downs depends on the particular substance involved and on the degree of adaption and addiction to it. Although this may vary from person to person and from substance to substance, the pattern of ups and downs remains consistent.

Remember Victor the taxi driver? His body was so adapted to fumes and auto emissions, as well as the city's many other air pollutants, that he became addicted to them. After he returned home from his day's work he was lethargic. No matter how much rest he got, he constantly complained that he was exhausted. He had no energy. He suffered from recurring respiratory infections, anxiety, and even depression. After much pleading, his wife finally convinced him to leave the city and go away for a much needed vacation at the seashore.

"It was an expensive trip, and I really didn't want to go," Victor said. "The only reason I went was to humor my wife and to please the kids, but it turned out that I had a wonderful time. I forgot how much fun the beach could be. I got out in the sunlight. I fished and surfed, and I felt better than I'd been feeling for a long time."

Once he was removed from the chemicals he had been enduring, his symptoms were unmasked. Unfortunately, as soon as he returned to work he became violently ill.

"I must have picked up a bug while we were away on our vacation," he insisted. "After a few hours at work I could barely breathe. I started coughing and choking. I had a headache and I was aching all over. I figured I had the flu. I went home and went to bed. The next day it was even worse. But what are you going to do? You can't give in and stay home. You have to go to work and earn a living for your family. I was miserable, but I managed to drag myself around for a few days. After a while I got over it, and I was fine."

Victor was not as fine as he thought. What really happened was that his return to work subjected him to the same chemicals that were making him sick in the first place. In his unmasked state, he returned to his original sensitivity and became ill. After several days of exposure, he readapted.

In our complex civilization, we are subject to so many different chemicals that it is possible that different chemicals can cause the same person to be in different stages of stimulation and withdrawal at the same time. When these stages overlap it is difficult to determine cause-and-effect relationships.

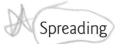 Spreading

Spreading turns multiple chemical sensitivity into a progressive disease in which the effects can spread from one part of the body to another. Someone whose original exposure caused severe respiratory problems may develop stomach problems, skin problems, difficulty concentrating, or any number of other difficulties.

In addition, once a person is sensitized to one chemical, the sensitivity can spread to include other chemicals. A person who was originally injured by a pesticide may eventually find that reactions are triggered by the smell of perfumed soap, certain foods, the formaldehyde used in building construction, or something as seemingly innocuous as the ink in the morning newspaper. After that happens, repeat exposures reduce the body's tolerance level. The body becomes more easily reactive to more and more chemicals at lower and lower levels until it finally reaches the point where the person is sick all the time.

Some people will develop increased sensitivity to multiple triggering agents, while others will have one isolated organ involved in their disease process for years. The disease only spreads to other organs as their resistance mechanisms break down. This kind of spreading from one organ to another or to multiple organs enables the progression of hypersensitivity and the eventual onset of specific diseases.

Spreading may occur because of a failure of the body's detoxification mechanisms: oxidation, reduction, degradation, and conjugation. It may be brought about by toxic overload, or it may occur because of the depletion of the enzyme or coenzyme's nutrient fuels, such as zinc, magnesium, all B vitamins, amino acid, or fatty acid. This depletion may account for an increasing inability to detoxify and respond appropriately. Various organs may be damaged, allowing previously excluded toxic and nontoxic substances to penetrate to areas that increase the risk of harm.

Switching

Switching makes this disease difficult to treat. A treatment may solve one problem, but unless the true source of symptoms is discovered and the offending pollutant eliminated, the disease may manifest itself somewhere else in the body and a completely new set of symptoms may crop up in a different organ or system.

This usually occurs immediately, but it may occur over a long period of time. The response to the pollutant will simply switch from one place to another. Sinusitis may be cleared by medication, but unless the chemical that caused it is eliminated, the person may later develop arthritis. Colitis may be cleared only for cystitis to develop. This lifelong progression of disease does not have to occur if the switch phenomenon is recognized. A person who sprays pesticides in his home may find himself visiting a neurologist with complaints of headaches, a rheumatologist with symptoms of arthritis, and a dermatologist with complaints of sudden acne, rash, or skin lesions. The patient as well as all the physicians may fail to recognize that these seemingly unrelated symptoms in different parts of the body are part of a larger pattern that needs further investigation. When the symptoms of each illness are treated separately, the whole person and his or her environment may be completely ignored. We ignore the whole person at our peril. At the heart of the human ecosystem is the immune system, a self-regulating mechanism that protects the body from invasion. Commonly, the symptoms are those of behavioral changes such as mood swings or even irrational behavior, respiratory and nasal congestion, skin rashes, and generalized fatigue. The spectrum of the syndrome ranges from slight, annoying symptoms all the way to severe disability.

Summary

Multiple chemical sensitivity is an insidious disease that affects multiple body systems, that has multiple symptoms, and that is caused by reactions to a wide variety of pollutants.

Although nobody can precisely pinpoint all its possible causes, multiple chemical sensitivity occurs when the body becomes unable to cope with the chemical overload of our environment and begins overreacting to what we consider common, everyday chemicals.

The symptoms and diseases caused by chemical exposures involve any and all parts of the body. Virtually every sickness known to general medicine or psychiatry can result from chemical exposure. In fact, a person can suffer from so many sicknesses that are so diverse, they can seem to be unbelievable. More than that, the frequent appearance of new symptoms during de-adaptation and re-exposure can make it even more difficult to recognize this disease for what it is. The following list summarizes the basic facts about multiple chemical sensitivity.

1. Biochemical individuality may include a genetic predisposition to sensitivity.

2. Poor diet and compromised nutrition can contribute to sensitivity.

3. The total body load at the time of exposure may include stress, toxins, infection, and previous exposures that were ignored, as well as other factors.

4. Induction, either as a high-level exposure or continuous low-level exposures to various substances, causes sensitization to a wide range of environmental agents.

5. Triggering can be brought on by exposure to the same chemicals that started the illness or by exposure to different chemicals altogether. Triggers can be lower levels of exposure than those in the original induction.

6. Masking, or adaptation, which can lead to addiction, may occur with continued exposures.

7. Bipolarity: In the adapted state the body may be stimulated by the offending substance, creating a high period. Continued exposures will cause the stimulatory phase to recede, and a down period will set in.

8. Spreading: A sensitivity to other, often chemically dissimilar, substances may trigger a different constellation of symptoms for each substance.

9. Switching: Treatment for one problem can be effective, but a completely new set of symptoms may begin in a completely different organ or system of the body. When this happens, the response to the pollutant has simply switched from one place to another.

10. Disability: If left untreated, sensitivity can lead to disease of specific organs, disability, and even death.

3

Pollution and Multiple Chemical Sensitivity

THE FABRIC OF our environment was woven in a delicate and harmonious balance that sustained the world and all the creatures in it. Even the worst natural disasters did little to threaten the overall delicate balance of life. For countless centuries, the Nile River overflowed its banks each year, depositing rich silt along its shores, transforming that long narrow strip of earth into fertile farmland where people could forge a stable civilization in an area that was primarily desert. Violent upheavals in the crust of the earth pushed land masses to the surface of the oceans, creating islands where people and animals could thrive. Even raging forest fires that swept across vast acreage burned away choking undergrowth, allowing young trees to find their place under the sun.

Primitive people who lived in close contact with their natural surroundings were careful to respect the harmony of Mother Earth and Father Sky. They believed everything in the world was carefully interconnected. Ireland's early Celts believed their forests and rivers possessed magical powers. The earliest Hebrews thanked God for every bountiful harvest. North American tribes believed the highest tribute to the Great Spirit was to leave no footprint in the path to disturb the tranquillity between what is, what was, and what will come again.

Progress in science and technology has allowed us to make drastic changes in our surroundings. In fact, the changes we have made since the Industrial Revolution have been more dramatic than those of all the centuries that came before. Our grandparents rode horse-drawn wagons to the market. We ride rockets to the moon.

Since the beginning of the Industrial Revolution, we have seen a dramatic change in attitudes as well as in technology. We have become ignorant, careless, and even willful in altering our delicately balanced surroundings. In doing so we have exposed ourselves to poisons our ancestors never imagined.

Whether we live in the nation's largest cities or in its hidden hollows, harmful chemical pollutants are released into the environment we eat, drink, breathe, and live in. We have bombarded our air, water, and land with increasing numbers of new chemicals. Sixty to eighty thousand chemicals are in common use with more developed every year. Each of these may have been designed to be beneficial, and many of them may be individually harmless, but in certain combinations, even in very low concentrations, they can become toxic. Nobody really understands what the long-term effects of a single new chemical will be, certainly not the effects of that chemical in combination with others, even in combination with other chemicals that by themselves are perfectly safe.

To make matters worse, we eat processed foods in which many of the nutrients have been destroyed. Both intentionally and unintentionally, we have refined away much of the nutritional value of the food we eat and replaced it with artificial colorings and flavorings, stabilizers, conditioners, and preservatives.

Our food supply has been compromised. Hormones fed to farm animals affect the way our children develop. Pesticides and fertilizers work their way into the ground and change the nature of the soil in which we grow our food. These chemicals as well as chemical additives become part of the foods we eat during processing, handling, and storage.

The water we drink is also polluted. Chemicals contaminate the lakes and rivers that supply our drinking water. Examination of our ground water has revealed low levels of hundreds of toxic chemicals. Extensive contamination of drinking water with allegedly low levels of synthetic pollutants is not harmless and should not be taken lightly. Toxic chemicals found in public water supplies include pesticides, herbicides, industrial solvents, and polychlorinated biphenyls. Mercury, zinc, and arsenic in the water are poisonous, and they are building to dangerous levels in our bodies. Slow damage to the body from the accumulated burden of these toxins becomes part of the problem of chronic illness. The incidence of many chronic diseases may be associated with the lack of purity in our water and air.

The three major sources of water pollution are city sewage, agricultural wastes, and industrial wastes. Agricultural wastes, including those from livestock, contain some of our most toxic substances. Nitrates in water, usually derived from agricultural fertilizers, pose an immediate threat to children under three months of age and a continuing threat to the rest of us. Pesticides, herbicides, fertilizers, and farm runoff collect in rivers, lakes, and ground water. Over one-half of the total volume of industrial wastes in the world's developed nations comes from paper mills, organic chemical manufacturing plants, petroleum companies, and steel manufacturing. The major pollutants are chemical byproducts, oil, grease, radioactive waste, and heat.

Inappropriately disposed of and improperly sealed, deadly materials have been accumulating in our waste dumps and landfills, slowly seeping out to contaminate our ground water. One high-profile example of water contamination that has captured public attention occurred in Times Beach, Missouri, where winter floods flushed out dioxin-contaminated oil that was used twenty years before. Incidents have also been recorded in Niagara's Love Canal Area; Waterbury, Connecticut; and Middleboro, Kentucky. Everywhere we live, lower-profile examples of contamination surround us.

Chemicals are intentionally added to our drinking water to protect us from infectious diseases. The interaction of chlorine with organic material can produce a toxic chemical combination. There are tested and proven alternatives to treating water with chlorine. For example, ozone has been used in Europe for years.

Many chemicals may appear to be inconsequential when tested individually, but when they are combined, their consequences multiply at an alarming rate. It might be reasonable to expect that chemical combinations are additive, so that the results of combining two chemicals would equal the effects of both chemicals. The unfortunate truth is that this is often not the case. Rather than gaining the beneficial results of each chemical, the chemicals combine to produce an entirely different result than was originally desired. When such chemical reactions occur, the results can be staggering.

When we discuss pollution, the first images that come to mind are tall industrial smokestacks belching dark smoke clouds into the clear blue sky until the sky becomes a muddy brown, until our cities become overhung with a miasma of murky haze. The very air we breathe is contaminated by chemical emissions that can travel over vast areas, so that we absorb fine particles. But we know that our oceans wash up globs of oil that may have been carelessly jettisoned or accidentally released at sea by monster tankers. Every tide fills our beaches with solid wastes, the discards of modern life. Industrial waste has been discharged into our waters until the blue waters turned black. The shores of our rivers and lakes have been darkened with decaying bodies of dead fish, unable to survive.

Although many of our laws and inspection agencies may still be considered controversial, improved environmental laws and advanced protective technology have improved environmental poisoning to a considerable extent. In many places steps have been taken to change the destruction of our surroundings.

Adaptation is a survival mechanism that unfortunately also makes warning signals disappear. A person adapts to constant toxic exposure in order to survive but, at the same time, suffers a long-term decrease in efficient functioning and perhaps longevity. Because of adaptation or tolerance, the patient's total body load may continue to increase while undetected because the perception of a cause-and-effect relationship has been lost.

With no warning symptoms, repeated exposures may continue and cause damage to the immune and enzyme detoxification systems. The eventual result of continued toxic exposure over a period of days, weeks, months, and years is end-organ failure.

Even though the future is far from secure, more stringent environmental laws and increased public awareness have had certain positive, concrete results. The pollution of our environment can be turned around. Once it was nearly dead, but now the Hudson River above New York City is returning to life. The Thames River above London again enjoys a viable population of fish. Lake Erie was once so polluted that its water was thick with muck, beaches were closed, and decaying fish and algae rotted on its shores; but it, too, is coming back to life. Air control standards put filters on those smokestacks so that the sky in many cities no longer drips brown soot.

In 1987, twenty-three nations signed the Montreal protocol, agreeing to gradually phase out the manufacture and use of ozone-destroying industrial compounds containing chlorine and fluorine. The most common of these included chlorofluorocarbons (CFCs), halons, and chlorine-based solvents used as refrigerants, cleaning agents, spray propellants, foams, and fire extinguishers. For the first time, measurements recently indicated that levels of many of these ozone-destroying chemicals are declining in the atmosphere. If this decline can continue for at least a decade, there is hope that the precious ozone layer can recover.

Evidence shows that the thousands of drugs, pesticides, and other pollutants in our environment remain stored in our bodies long after we are first exposed to them. Chemicals stored in the body pose a serious threat to both physical and mental health.

Our bodies are equipped with various natural detoxification systems, but we were hardly designed to cope with the heavy loads that currently attack us. Since our bodies have no previous experience with these new chemicals, they are not equipped to break them down or to eliminate them. The changing content of our diets in combination with the extensive absorption of chemicals may have destined many people to experience a kind of internal pollution.

Health depends on a balance of both external and internal environmental forces. In the normal detoxification process, the healthy body neutralizes the effect of specific pollutants and manages to balance itself. It is possible that a person whose body cannot handle the unnaturally large numbers of chemicals attacking its limited detoxification systems may develop chemical sensitivity syndrome.

This assortment of diseases comes about because of an overload that alters the body's natural balance. Overwhelmed by vast numbers of chemicals, even the healthiest person can develop a combination of altered body metabolism, enzyme dysfunction, nutritional deficiencies, and hormonal imbalances that may result in a dramatically lowered resistance threshold. This makes it impossible for the body to cope with both the natural and unnatural environments. When a deluge of chemicals overwhelms the body's defense systems, we become sick and unable to function.

Chemical sensitivity is spreading to epidemic proportions, with more and more people becoming sick as their bodies are unable to cope with the toxic overload. Chemicals like formaldehyde, toluene, xylene, benzene, vinyl chloride, trichlorethane, styrene, and phthalates are not easy to detect when they are absorbed by the body over extended periods of time. Long-term exposure can build up silently until the body becomes overburdened. When that happens the victim of chemical poisoning may develop a great many symptoms in a many different organ systems.

Symptoms vary from one person to the next. Some symptoms can even appear to be mental problems. These might include confusion, memory loss, irritability, depression, or anxiety. Some people may find that they are frequently dizzy or they may describe the "spacy" sensation of not quite being in control. Some people will lose their ability to concentrate. Some will develop severe headaches, recurrent infections, irritable bowel syndrome, joint aches, or muscle pains. Others may suffer from constant fatigue that no amount of rest can cure. The symptoms can involve so many different parts of the body and vary so greatly that they may appear to be entirely unrelated.

All people have individual strengths and weaknesses. Some may be less sensitive to the toxic environment than others. Although not everyone will suffer from chemical sensitivity in the same way or to the same degree, those who are unfortunate enough to develop multiple chemical sensitivity are sounding the alarm, warning the rest of us that, even though we may not be suffering at this moment, our health is seriously at risk from invisible pollution.

It would be foolish to suggest we abandon the progress that makes it possible for constantly increasing numbers of people to survive and to enjoy an improved standard of living. Nobody would reasonably advocate that we all return to scratching out a meager subsistence in primitive conditions. What is sane, sensible, and entirely reasonable is that responsible means of protecting the environment become a required part of production to provide for the health of our world.

4

Iris's Story

WE'VE ALL BEEN SICK. Everybody knows how you get sick. You wake up in the morning feeling out of sorts. Your eyes are red and itchy. Your stomach flutters. By noon you find that you've developed the sniffles. By dinner time your nose is red, your throat is raw, and your fever has you running hot and cold. You visit the doctor, you take your medicine, you stay in bed, and ten days later you feel better. Sickness is that simple. Or is it?

Iris will tell you quite another story. "Living with multiple chemical sensitivity is nothing better than a life of hell," she said. "You can't go where you want to go, you can't work at what you want to do or even at what you were trained to do. You can't wear the kind of clothing you want to wear. Friendships are affected. Your whole life is affected. Relationships break up when the partners don't understand what's going on, why you're suddenly so sickly, why you're suddenly acting crazy, why everything bothers you, why you can't go out and do things like a normal person. Every time I walk through my door, I'm walking outside in fear because I know something bad is going to happen to me. No matter how careful I am, I'm going to be subjected to one of the things that causes me to react, and I'm likely to come home sick and have to go to bed for days."

Iris wasn't always sick. She didn't always live with the fear of stepping outside her house. Her trouble started while she was working for a bank that was in the process of remodeling its offices. All the employees were delighted with the proposed renovations, with the new look, and with the prospect of spending their days working in more cheerful surroundings. Unfortunately, so many harmful chemicals were involved in the massive renovation that Iris will never be entirely sure which had the most toxic effect on her body and on her life.

"The first thing the workmen did when they started the remodeling project was to move all the new carpet squares onto my floor, so that I was in close contact with them all day," she said. Since it was one of those inconveniences one might expect during a major remodeling project, she didn't see any reason to complain. In fact, she didn't even think much about it. "At the same time, they started painting with oil-based paints. I started to experience difficulty the first time they opened a can of oil paint, but I didn't really know what was happening to me. I knew the solvents smelled bad. I knew that the constant smell gave me what I thought was a little headache, and it made me feel sick to my stomach, but a smell is only a smell. Paint is such a normal part of everyday life I was sure it couldn't hurt me. I just stayed where I was and continued working. After a while, I got accustomed to the smell so that I didn't really smell it anymore. I was too busy with the upset stomach and the headache to worry about something as simple as a smell."

Always an active person who was involved in community activities, Iris attended a political fund-raiser after work that day. She knew something was seriously wrong because even though she had always been lively and alert she found herself strangely subdued that evening. She was in the company of a great many people. They were her friends and associates, but they might as well have been total strangers. She was unable to reach out to them. She found herself unable to communicate with people or with her surroundings. She suddenly found that she was completely unable to take in information, to process it appropriately, or to respond in a reasonable manner.

"I had trouble putting my thoughts together," she said. "I was confused and I was having trouble simply trying to talk. I'm a talker. Anyone who knows me would know that's not like me. That's not something I'd ever had trouble doing before. When I did try to talk, my words came out garbled. No matter how hard I tried, my words didn't come out right. I was quiet all evening, hoping no one would notice."

The next morning she was so sick she couldn't get out of bed. She felt as though she was paralyzed. Her body would not move. She summoned enough strength to call in sick and remained in bed for two days. On the third day she was finally able to get up and to drag herself to work. Although she felt sicker as the day progressed, she completed her work. She managed to survive the week but she was so sick she remained in bed during the weekend. "After I stayed at home for several days I started to feel better, but when I went to work and was subjected to those construction materials I would get sicker and sicker," she said.

Convinced that she was suffering from a virus or from some related discomfort that would soon go away, Iris did everything possible to cope with her mysterious ailment. She continued to go to her job, although she had to force herself to get out of bed in the morning. She had to force herself to dress and to drive her car. Her energy abandoned her. Some days she was so exhausted she went home at noon and took a brief but much-needed nap during her lunch hour. Some days she was so weak she had to leave work early. On the occasions when she could find the strength to work a full day, she would go directly home and fall into bed, unable to do another thing. When she did not improve after a month had passed, she called her doctor. "Something's wrong," she told him. "I feel as though I'm dying."

Her family doctor believed she was having an allergic reaction to the products that were used in the bank's renovation and assured her she would soon be able to return to work and to her normal schedule. He told her that as soon as the renovation was completed she would be fine again.

Luckily, the renovations were temporarily shut down. The contractors were absent, and their supplies were not used. Everything seemed to be fine, at least during that short time. She thought she was improving and dared to hope that her life and health would return to normal.

Immediately after the contractors returned and resumed painting, Iris began to experience breathing problems. She then developed asthma, which she had never had before. Her symptoms became so severe she was hospitalized. When she was discharged from the hospital and returned home, she remained in bed for two weeks. Then, determined that she would not to lose her job, she went back to work.

"When I was away from the bank for a couple of weeks I felt better, but as soon as I returned I started to get sick again. Before long I was gasping for air," she said. "I felt as though I was drowning, but there was no water. I was drowning in air. That was when I realized I could not go back there. As much as I loved my job, I simply could not go back.

While I was out of work, my case was turned over to Workman's Compensation. They assigned me to a doctor who was supposed to be an environmental doctor. If he was an environmental doctor, he should have understood my problems more completely than he did. I continued to see him for nine months. He didn't really harm me, but he didn't help me much either. I now believe that because he worked for Workman's Compensation the things he wrote up on his medical evaluation were not as thorough as they should have been. In his evaluation, he said I didn't have a problem, so I was released with no compensation for anything. By the time this happened I had become unbearably sick, and I was unable to work. I was forced to sue Workman's Comp. to try to get some much-needed monetary compensation."

Iris was reluctant to enter into a legal suit, but she had no choice. "I had to give a deposition," she said. "It took all day to do it, and the attorneys were horrible to me, just horrible. They were unbelievably rude. They treated me as though I was nuts. I've never been treated like that before. I've never been through anything like that in my life. It depressed me so badly that I don't even remember half of what I said. Although I didn't realize what was happening to me until after I was seriously affected, I was apparently having problems with the room where the deposition was taking place. This happens sometimes to people with multiple chemical sensitivities. Before you realize what's happening to you, you can find yourself in serious trouble."

The attorneys subjected Iris to five-and-a-half hours of interrogation, eroding her confidence, sapping her strength, wearing her down until she began to cry. "When I reached that point I just stood up and walked out of the room and said, 'I can't take this any more.'"

Her attorney finally understood what was happening. "He told them that in the future they could have two hours of my time maximum and not one minute more. They agreed to that, but of course the Workman's Compensation was denied."

In the two years since she suffered her first major exposure, Iris has gone from being an active, employed, productive, independent person to becoming a semirecluse.

"I have been accepted for Social Security Disability," she explained. "I never knew something like this would happen to me. I've always worked hard and earned my own way. I've always been active in my community, helping other people who needed help. It's embarrassing for me to have to accept this help, but I have no choice. I can't work. I'm single. I have to have some way to live. It took me more than a year to get the Social Security Disability, and I know that I was fortunate at that since most people have to wait two to three years or more until they're granted a hearing, and it's unusual for them to accept multiple chemical sensitivity as a disability. For the first time I began to understand why you see so many street people these days. When I see those poor people I wonder how many of them are suffering from something like this and are undiagnosed and unable to get help."

Iris spent a desperate year trying to find medical help. "I knew that if I was ever going to improve, I had to find a doctor who could help me. I knew there had to be someone out there who understood what was wrong with me, but I didn't know who it might be. I didn't know where to go. Everyone I knew had a suggestion for me, but most of the suggestions they offered turned out to be useless. The Workman's Compensation doctor didn't help me at all. My family doctor knew it was something more than he could handle so he sent me to an allergist. The allergist then sent me to a diagnostic facility where I had a truly horrible experience with a doctor who didn't understand anything at all about what I was going through.

"After doing all these long, painful, and expensive tests, he realized that I had problems, and he knew I had really bad problems but he thought my problems were all in my head. He actually had the nerve to tell me he thought my problems would not be as bad if I had a man in my life. It was devastating! I had driven for five hours to get to the diagnostic facility. I'd had to spend the night in a hotel room which I could not afford. I underwent all those tests. I worried about the results. I was facing a five-hour drive back home alone, and that was all he had to say to me? A man in my life? I came home from that trip exhausted and sick. I walked through the door to my house and broke down and cried.

"I was having trouble traveling, and I realized I couldn't go on chasing all these doctors from one office to the next, from one city to the next. I was too sick to go out and find another doctor. After that experience I decided I would not see another doctor without first interviewing him on the phone."

Meanwhile, Iris's health continued to deteriorate. She awakened some mornings feeling as though she did not have enough strength to make it through the day. She'd take her shower, read the newspaper, and become so sick she would be forced to return to bed. "I would be totally fatigued. I would be so sleepy I would be out of it for hours," she said.

After several months of suffering she came to understand that it was the printer's ink in the daily newspaper that was making her sick. She was leafing through a health magazine when she found an ad offering reading bags for multiple chemical sensitivity patients. In the desperate hope that this product would allow her to read books as well as newspapers again, she impulsively called the long distance number listed in the ad.

"I found myself talking with a doctor and his wife who had started a company that offered products to help people like me. They had such items as safe soaps, safe shampoo, safe household cleaning supplies, as well as reading bags for multiple chemical sensitivity patients. They also offered a reading box, but it was very expensive and I couldn't afford it. In our conversation, the doctor told me that his wife also suffered from multiple chemical sensitivity. As they started searching for products that would make her life more comfortable, they eventually became involved with selling these products to help other people."

Even though the long-distance call was an expense Iris could not very well afford in her reduced financial situation, she was so delighted to have found someone who understood her problems, she and the stranger at the other end of the line talked for quite a long time. "I can't tell you what a comfort it was to speak with someone who understood me, someone who knew what I was going through. When I told him about my terrible experiences trying to find a physician who knew what was wrong with me, he immediately recommended Dr. Edelson. He said, 'I want you to do this first thing in the morning. Don't wait. Do it as soon as you get up. Don't hesitate, but call Dr. Edelson and tell him what's been happening to you. I think he's going to help you.' "

By this time Iris was so discouraged she honestly didn't believe anyone or anything could help her, but she called the Environmental and Preventive Health Center of Atlanta and requested a telephone interview with Dr. Edelson.

"I was too sick to continue the hopeless march from doctor to doctor. I didn't know what else I could do, or even what else I should do, but I knew that seeing all these doctors was hurting me more than it was helping me and I couldn't do it anymore. The only thing that made any sense was for me to talk to Dr. Edelson before I made the effort to see him," she explained. "We talked on the phone for more than an hour. He didn't talk down to me, and he certainly didn't try to tell me my sickness was all in my head. He even sent me a patient list of people he was treating for different things, including multiple chemical sensitivity. They were people who had problems like mine. I telephoned quite a few of these people before I decided to set up an appointment with him. After all my bad experiences, I had to be convinced this doctor would really understand my problems. You don't find doctors in this specialty unless they have been faced with the reality of these problems.

"Before you even go into Dr. Edelson's office, his staff tells you not to wear perfume, not to wear anything that has a scent to it, and to be careful of how you wash the clothes you're going to wear when you come in for your office visit. I didn't understand all of these precautions. They sounded pretty strange to me at first, but I did what they told me to do. I can understand them now. I have found myself in other doctor's offices where I had to get up and ask the nurse if I could wait in another room because the person beside me had used fabric softener when washing her clothes. Most people wouldn't smell it, or if they did smell it they would think it was a pleasant smell. Unfortunately, it's one of those triggers that causes me to react badly.

"In spite of all these precautions, I actually suffered an attack several months later while I was in Dr. Edelson's office. Shortly before I arrived there I must have been exposed to something that triggered my illness. When I realized what was happening, I went up to the nurse and told her I was in trouble. She could see that I was going into a bad reaction to something. That day Dr. Edelson sat and held my hand for four or five hours off and on while he gave me oxygen and an IV that was full of nutrients. He had to order a ceramic oxygen mask for me because I can't even use standard plastic tubing because I was so sensitive to it. This ceramic mask makes it much easier for me to be able to use the oxygen, which helps me with my breathing and with my joint pain."

Since her illness began, every aspect of Iris's life has changed. She uses air purifiers in her house. She uses a water purifier. She even has an air purifier that she uses in her car. Unfortunately, she can't accept anything new in her surroundings. She even has to be careful of the clothes she wears.

"Some clothes, particularly permanent press clothes, have formaldehyde right in the cloth," she explained. "I can develop problems with dyes and with synthetic materials, so I wear mostly natural cotton clothing. Even so, I have difficulty wearing things that have been dry cleaned. I even have difficulty being near people whose clothes have been dry cleaned. I can't be around people who use cosmetics. I can smell scented laundry detergent in other people's clothes and it will make me sick."

She's also had some terrible difficulties in beauty shops. "I have to be very careful around hair spray, shampoo, everything like that," Iris said. "I decided to cut my long hair short and wear it straight because I know that I can never have another perm. When I absolutely have to have a haircut, I put it off as long as I can because I know how dangerous it can be for me to go into the beauty shop. When I can't put it off any longer, I try to go on days that aren't busy. I try to make my appointment first thing in the morning when the shop is not yet filled with all the smells of someone else having color put on her hair or having a perm put in her hair. All those chemicals are offensive now, and they are dangerous to me."

The simple, everyday act of going to a mall or shopping center is all but impossible for Iris. If she must make a purchase, she decides on a plan of attack, maps out the quickest way to get in and out of the store, and hurries to get her shopping done. The mall's various stores with all the variety of clothing dyes and synthetic fabrics are painful for her to endure. This marks a complete change in lifestyle for a woman who once loved to shop. When she was working, she made it a practice to walk the mall every day during her lunch hour as a way to get her exercise. "I can't do that anymore," she said sadly, "If I tried to walk the mall the way I used to do, I would be sick by the time I left."

Of course, Iris wasn't always sick. "I wasn't like this before this happened. I had a few allergies, and I had taken allergy shots for a few years. Occasionally, if someone was wearing too much perfume I would find it offensive, but I didn't think that was unusual because when someone wears too much perfume everybody finds it offensive. Since this happened and I became sick, perfumes affect me so badly that someone can just walk past me and I'll start having bronchial spasms and breathing problems, I'll feel spacy and disoriented, all those things that go with an asthma attack. Of course, you can ask your friends not to wear perfume and they'll accommodate you, but sometimes they don't remember or they don't understand. Sometimes they'll say, 'I didn't put anything on,' and that might be true, but they still have scent remaining on their clothes from the last time they wore perfume."

One night she was enjoying dinner with some friends when she started to be uncomfortable. It felt as though she was beginning to have an asthma attack. She realized that one of her dinner companions "smelled as though he had poured a bottle of cologne on himself." She rushed home, gasping for breath before the full attack came over her. Following an attack, she usually becomes nauseated. She develops joint pain, followed by a migraine headache.

"I have prepared a chemically safe oasis inside my house where I can retreat when I've had a particularly bad chemical affront. I'll have to stay there in my safe, purified environment for days and days trying to get well. But as soon as I start to feel a little bit better, or when I can't stand being in there any longer, I'll go out somewhere and try to live my life like a normal person. I may go out to dinner with friends, I may go visit a friend's house, or I'll try to go to a meeting or to a movie. This can cause more problems, and it takes me two to three weeks to get over it. I have chronic fatigue and chronic pain. Dr. Edelson tells me I need to stay out of those environments. I know he's right. I know it's foolish of me, but I resent it. If I can't go out to a restaurant for an occasional dinner, if I can't visit friends, I'm not living a normal life, and I resent not being able to live something close to a normal life. I can't stay home all the time and become a vegetable! I try to be careful about where I go."

Iris described a sickness that can change a normal life: "It goes from simple to a place where every phase of your life is affected," she said, and her voice was the voice of experience.

5

Who Is at Risk?

OUR AIR, our water, and our food supplies have become more polluted and more comprehensively filled with synthetic chemicals. These changes have come about so quickly it has been impossible for our bodies to adjust to the host of new chemicals and combinations of chemicals that have intentionally or unintentionally been added to our environment. The resulting environmental damage causes people to become sick in ever-increasing numbers with a variety of symptoms that may affect any and all of the body's systems.

As a species, human beings have been remarkably able to cope with change during the long centuries of our existence in both recorded and unrecorded time. Multiple chemical sensitivity is developing so rapidly because we are simply not equipped to change quickly enough to accommodate the speed of the chemical changes that are taking place in our environment. Although we may be taller and have bigger feet, our bodies are basically the same as those of our ancestors who lived thousands of years ago. The world we live in, however, is much different.

Everyone is at risk for exposure. However, four groups of people have been specifically identified as being at significant risk. They include industrial workers; people who work in "sick," or "tight," buildings, including school teachers and school children who work and attend classes in "sick" school buildings; people who live and work in chemically contaminated communities; and people who are at risk in the alleged safety of their own homes.

Industrial Workers

Industrial workers are subject to acute and chronic exposure to industrial chemicals. These are frequently men between the ages of twenty and sixty-five years of age.

People Who Work in "Sick" Buildings

Men and women who work in tight, or sick, buildings are subject to inadequate ventilation, which magnifies the effects of office supplies, tobacco smoke, pesticides, and gases released from synthetic construction materials and furnishings. Since a greater number of women are employed in office work, women are more frequently affected by sick buildings than are men. These women are frequently twenty to sixty-five years old and are office workers, teachers, and medical personnel.

School children are at significant risk when they attend classes in tight buildings. These are frequently the newer, more modern and energy-efficient school buildings that have been constructed since the 1970s or that have been renovated since that time. The children may come from every socioeconomic or cultural background and are prekindergarten through high school age.

People Who Live and Work in
Chemically Contaminated Communities

People of all ages who live and work in communities where air and water have been contaminated by chemicals are exposed through toxic waste sites, nearby agricultural spraying, ground water contamination, automobiles, trucks, and local industrial emissions. Children and infants may be the first to be affected by such exposure, and they may be the most severely affected, along with the elderly and pregnant women and their babies.

People in Their Homes

This is an extremely difficult group to isolate because their exposure comes from contaminated air inside their homes, contaminated water, consumer products, gases released from building materials, and drugs and pesticides. They are frequently women between the ages of thirty and fifty.

Some people who suffer from multiple chemical sensitivity will remember a single experience of high-level exposure. Others may suffer from continued low-level exposures that may continue to be unnoticed until serious damage has been done. The more symptoms the person suffers, the more systems of the body that are affected, and the more severely the many symptoms change in intensity, the stronger the suspicion of multiple chemical sensitivity.

When people who are as different as industrial workers and school children develop strikingly similar complaints and suffer from many of the same symptoms triggered by chemical exposure, it becomes obvious that the similarities of their physical problems and the history of their exposure is more than merely a coincidence.

6

What Is Environmental Medicine?

ENVIRONMENTAL MEDICINE is the study of the effects of our environment on our individual health. It includes the water we drink, the food we eat, the air we breathe, inhalants, biologicals, chemicals, metals, and our physical surroundings. It is based on the belief that chronic, constant, debilitating disease has biochemical causes, that these diseases may have an environmental trigger, and that they can be stopped.

The philosophy of environmental medicine teaches that the absence of diagnosable disease is not necessarily the equivalent of good health. True health is looking, feeling, and performing at optimum levels. Harmful chemicals make it impossible to enjoy optimum health because even when they are present only in small amounts they can seriously damage the human body. Chronic degenerative diseases are not and should not be an expected or acceptable part of life.

Many of the illnesses associated with a generally failing standard of health may be linked to the harmful effects of taking foreign substances into the body either voluntarily or involuntarily during the normal course of everyday life. Environmental medicine carefully considers all those things that may be taken into the body. These include things we may eat, drink, breathe, or absorb through the skin.

Many chemical antigens may cause a primary allergic response. They are not dispelled from the body but remain inside over a long period of time, acting as continual irritants. The illnesses that result from this poisonous storage and the toll it takes on our bodies can be long term. Once a person is sensitized by a harmful substance, future exposure to the same substance or to a wide range of varying substances can lead to dangerous and debilitating illness.

We sometimes tend to think environmental illness happens all at once because we usually become aware of it all at once, but the truth is that it is not a sudden, acute ailment. Just as a heart attack or arterial blockage may take years to develop, environmental illness also develops over time. It can take years to develop. It finally becomes critical when the body's immune and detoxication systems become so overloaded they can no longer cope with the damage environmental illness has caused and eventually collapse.

The continuous accumulation of harmful substances that cannot be disposed of by the body eventually leads to degenerative disease. Many factors have an effect on this development. Some of the factors may involve a person's heredity, his nutritional status at the time of exposure, alcohol and drug consumption, work environment, home environment, food, hypersensitivities, inhalant allergies, and even Candida (yeast) related conditions. These damaging substances are made even more dangerous when combined with that person's specific metabolic and nutritional deficiencies.

Environmental medicine is a relatively new area in the practice of medicine. It deals with sickness that is preventable. It attempts to forestall illness by helping the body to help itself. This often involves both traditional and complementary methods of medical care to enhance and strengthen the body's own defenses.

Who Are the Doctors Who Practice Environmental Medicine?

Doctors who practice environmental and preventive medicine are state-licensed physicians with backgrounds in such diverse specialties as internal medicine, pediatrics, allergy, gynecology, psychiatry, surgery, and other areas.

Many of them have developed holistic philosophies and consider their patients to be whole people rather than a series of malfunctioning body parts in need of technical repairs. They are biochemically oriented and nutritionally minded. They have chosen to follow an ongoing, enlightened, and innovative approach to their personal educations after they have completed medical training. They have expanded their expertise to state-of-the-art innovative medicine that they use in addition to traditional contemporary medical techniques. These doctors are both scientifically curious and deeply concerned about the people who come to them to seek their help.

Do They Use All the Modern Technology Currently Available to the Medical Profession?

Of course they use all the traditional tools available, including X-rays, blood work, advanced laboratory tests, and advanced diagnostic studies. However, since everything that happens in a person's life will affect that person's physical and emotional health, environmental physicians also employ detailed family and individual histories, which are gained through interviews and assessments. Health and personal histories are carefully documented in addition to the purely physical findings of intensive examination and testing.

Although technology is dramatically effective in pinpointing the specific health problems of specific body systems, it is seldom a substitute for the time that is spent listening carefully to what people have to say. When a person is left out of his own diagnosis, appropriate medical care may be seriously compromised. Both the patient and the physician are obliged to spend the considerable amount of time necessary to complete thorough interviews, but time spent in conversation can reveal significant information about a person's true state of health as well as the problems and background experiences that may have contributed to that state of health.

The sick person comes to the doctor complete with a functioning mind in addition to a somewhat malfunctioning body. He has hopes and fears. He comes to the doctor searching for optimism and empowerment to cope with sickness and with the very real difficulties of living through a complicated illness.

Is This Approach a New Idea?

The idea that a sick person is a full human being is certainly not new. Almost two thousand years ago, the ancient Greek Hippocrates considered precisely these ideas when he wrote: "All parts of the body which are destined for a definite use are kept in health and in the enjoyment of fair growth and of long youth by the fulfillment of that use and by their suitable exercise in the duty for which they were made." To this day, doctors of medicine swear to the Hippocratic oath, which was first proposed by this great thinker and healer. Among other things, it requires a physician to swear that he will always help the sick with all his knowledge and power, that he will supply no poison to anyone, that he will abstain from every evil use of the means and instrument of his art, and that he will always keep his patient's secrets.

In his treatise "The Aphorisms of Moses," the twelfth-century physician and scholar Moses Maimonides wrote, "May I never consider him [the patient] to be no more than merely a vessel of disease." Even at that early time, Maimonides advocated a holistic approach and counseled physicians to treat the whole patient, not merely a specific symptom. He wrote, "In consideration of the effects of psychic mood, it is generally acknowledged that the impact of mental suffering, agitation, and obstinacy is to impair mental activity and physical well-being."

He also advocated the rights of patients not to be subdued by a physician's paternalism. He thought that a physician was duty bound to offer the best possible medical advice, even when it might be contrary to his own or to his patient's personal belief system. It was the patient's responsibility to accept or to reject the advice the physician offered.

Maimonides wrote a treatise on asthma in 1190. In it he observed that people who are inclined toward asthma react strongly to certain irritants. Even at that early time, he prescribed a correct diet and treatments for mind, body, and spirit because he realized these things have a positive effect on asthmatics.

Will the Environmental Physician Understand a Patient Who Suffers from a Variety of Problems?

Even though you come into the office suffering from what might sound like a catalog of miseries, a good environmental physician understands that you are not exaggerating the extent of your sickness. She will trust that you are telling the truth about your suffering. People don't want to be sick. Your illness is real, and you are not simply looking for sympathy. You are not looking for relief from a job you may not enjoy or from life situations you do not find pleasant. Your sickness is not an expression of your unhappiness. Your sickness is not a way to blame your problems on outside forces. Your sickness is not a way to gain sympathy or to avoid responsibility. It is sickness. You want help; you want a way to relieve the symptoms of your illness.

A good environmental physician will never dismiss your concerns with such clichés as "it's only your nerves" and will not send you off to the psychiatrist or psychologist simply because you complain about a wide spectrum of symptoms.

Biochemical Individuality

Since each person is unique, the causes and symptoms of an illness in one person may prove to be completely different in another person. Environmental physicians are trained to recognize biochemical individuality. They know that unique patient profiles result from evaluating individual biochemistry, nutrition, and environments.

Since no two people are alike, everyone suffering from the same disease should not necessarily be subjected to the same treatment. Instead, treatment should be individualized to satisfy the particular needs of the particular person at a particular time. Individual recommendations are designed to achieve an optimum level of health.

Although he may not immediately be able to come up with instant simple answers for your particular complicated set of problems, an environmental physician will be painstakingly thorough in making evaluations and will work diligently to tailor a plan of treatment specifically for you.

The causes of environmental illnesses can be a mystery. When did your illness start? Where did your illness start? What is your illness doing to you? How are you affected by certain specific chemicals? What can be done to avoid your specific problems? Most environmental physicians are willing to take on the role of Sherlock Holmes, using every diagnostic aid and innovative approach that is currently available to help solve that mystery. These doctors don't mind doing detective work.

Who Are Their Patients?

Environmental physicians see people from every walk of life. They see people who are suffering from a wide variety of problems. They see people suffering from fatigue, lethargy, headaches, depression, anxiety, arthritis, abdominal difficulties, poor memory, impaired concentration, sexual difficulties, recurring infections, ringing in the ears, PMS, anorexia, bulimia, schizophrenia, mercury toxicity, eczema, allergies, colitis, irritable bowel syndrome, hyperactivity, and many other ailments. They see people who are suffering from many ailments at once, and they know that these ailments have a physical cause.

Diagnosis

The search for the environmental triggers that provoke symptoms and result in sickness focuses on chemical, nutritional, and biological incitants. Diagnoses for food allergies are based on tests like elimination diets, provocation-neutralization skin testing, and ALCAT food sensitivity testing. Diagnostic tests for low-level chemical exposure may include avoidance of incitants, provocation-neutralization tests, and "inhalation booth" challenges as well as tests like the ALCAT and Elisa–ACT.

Treatment

Treatments may include avoidance, neutralization, enzyme potentiated desensitization, nutrition, and detoxification. Enzyme potentiated desensitization is a technique that uses extremely small doses of allergens to attempt to desensitize the patient against his allergies. It can be a successful treatment that has dramatically helped many people.

Since your sickness is your personal possession, the responsibility for getting well must be your personal choice. Some of your treatment will involve making necessary changes in your way of living. Some of these changes may be drastic. Since drastic lifestyle changes can be extremely difficult, your doctor will help you and encourage you in making the appropriate choices and changes.

How Does the Environmental Physician Work with You?

Patients can and should contribute their own observations and insights when evaluating the status of their health. An environmental physician will encourage you to do so. Control lies with the patient as an intelligent, capable human being who is in need of help. The physician is not a puppeteer who pulls the strings and expects his patient to dance to the tune but a partner in achieving good health. A good environmental physician is a caring fellow human being, a coach who can encourage and inspire the lifestyle changes necessary to help you return to optimum health.

How Did Environmental Medicine Come About?

Immediately after World War II, the general public became painfully aware of the environmental causes of illness. The development of the atomic bomb left little doubt in anyone's imagination. The aftermath of the atomic bomb and the fear of radioactive fallout led people to think carefully about the nature of the food chain.

As horrible as the prospect of nuclear annihilation might have been, at least nuclear bombs falling from the sky and landing at ground zero were kind enough to kill their victims outright. The public heard horror stories about slow, painful deaths resulting from radioactive fallout, the concentration of nuclear matter in water, milk, meat, and vegetables grown in contaminated soil. People realized that radioactive fallout was not the only danger facing humankind. Interest in the environment and in the world around us began to grow.

Environmental illness was first observed in a patient by Theron G. Randolph, a board-certified allergist. He received his M.D. from the University of Michigan and his Allergy and Immunology Fellowship at Massachusetts General Hospital and Harvard University Medical School. He entered into private practice in Chicago, where he also served as Clinical Instructor in Allergy at Northwestern University Medical School.

During the 1940s and 1950s, he realized that not only foods but also certain chemicals might be causing symptoms in his patients and that people were getting sick because of changes in the environment. He began to publish papers about food allergies.

During his testimony before the National Food and Drug Administration, he became the first physician to recommend carefully labeling prepared food to include its specific ingredients. It wasn't until many years later that these changes were adopted so that we are now able to read clear, easily understandable, concise labels on all our packaged foods. Until that time we had no idea what was in the pre-pared food we were eating. Obviously, Randolph was ahead of his time.

Randolph also first described the concept of chemical sensitivity. In a much publicized case, he described the experiences of a patient whom he had been treating for combinations of rhinitis, asthma, headaches, unbearable fatigue, irritability, depression, widely changing weight gain and loss, and episodes where she would lose consciousness.

After careful observation and documentation of her episodes of sickness, he realized that each event was connected in some way to an exposure to gas, oil, coal, or their combustion products. When the woman was able to avoid these incitants, her condition improved. He began to observe and record the experiences of other patients who had similar complaints. They, too, improved when they were able to avoid specific items.

Randolph developed the first true understanding that it is not only foods but also the chemicals found in the environment that can cause an illness that is similar to allergy. He published a series of abstracts in the *Journal of Laboratory and Clinical Medicine* that documented allergic-type reactions to industrial solvents and liquid fuels, mosquito fogs and mists, motor exhausts, indoor utility gas and oil fumes, and coal or petrochemically derived additives in foods, drugs, and cosmetics. He also noted that environmental influences can affect emotional and behavioral activity in a demonstrable cause-and-effect way.

He developed a systematic approach to the study of how individuals respond to food and chemicals. His approach was to totally remove people from their environments and then to expose them separately to each food and to each chemical. By doing this he was able to discover the two-phased response now known as the adapted-and-withdrawal response.

In the 1950s Randolph adopted the term *clinical ecology* to describe his focus on environmentally induced illness. In 1960, Randolph and several other allergists founded the Society for Clinical Ecology and opened its doors to physicians who were interested or involved in environmental study. Over time, the specialty has evolved from simply addressing allergies to food or sensitivities to chemicals into several specialized categories.

The publication of Rachel Carson's book *Silent Spring* in 1962 brought the pending environmental disasters clearly into public focus. In her book she outlined the catastrophes facing the world as the result of the careless use of chemicals in the environment, including the deaths and potential extinction of large numbers of insects, animals, birds, fish, and other wildlife; the destruction of water sources; and the pollution of the land.

In the early 1970s, Dr. William Rea, a thoracic and cardiovascular surgeon, began having attacks of dizziness and suffering from unexplained flulike symptoms. He saw a physician who diagnosed an ecological illness. The diagnosis and treatment led to a change in the direction of Rea's life work. He began to specialize in the treatment of patients who suffered similar illnesses and has led scientific development of this field. He founded the Environmental Health Center of Dallas. His work helped develop environmental medicine to maturity.

In 1982, Dr. Rea, Dr. Randolph, and Dr. Doris Rapp, world leaders in clinical ecology, gave a series of lectures on the effects of the environment on health in Germany and in England.

In 1987, Dr. Rea was awarded the Jonathan Forman Gold Medal Award by the American Academy of Environmental Medicine. In 1988, he was named to the world's first professorial chair of environmental medicine at the Robens Institute of Toxicology at the University of Surrey in Guildford, England. In 1993, he was awarded the Herbert J. Rinkel Award by the American Academy of Environmental Medicine. He serves on the board of directors of both the American Academy of Environmental Medicine and the American Environmental Health Foundation.

In 1985, the Society for Clinical Ecology changed its name to the American Academy of Environmental Medicine. Membership has grown to more than seven hundred physicians. An examination leading to certification in environmental medicine is offered.

In 1987, Mark Cullen, Professor of Medicine and Epidemiology at Yale University Medical School, established seven major diagnostic features of environmental illness, making it easier to diagnose.

Environmental medicine will meet the challenges of the twenty-first century with vision and energy, state-of-the-art diagnostic studies, technological advancement, and affirmation of the dignity of the individual. The latest in medical technology combined with a compassionate human face is needed now more than ever as we go forward into the new millennium.

7

Judith's Story

EVEN THOUGH JUDITH has earned degrees in both counseling and psychology and has worked as a physician's assistant, she didn't know what was happening to her when she got sick. All she knew was that she couldn't find help for her various ailments. "I should have known better, but I didn't realize what was wrong with me at the time," she said. "I did know that while I was working at a medical facility I was exposed to quite a lot of chemicals. What finally put me over the edge was a gas leak, which compromised my immune system." She began to develop symptoms that were so diverse and were located in so many different parts of her body that, even with her medical background, it did not occur to her that they might possibly be related.

"When my nose stopped up I thought I had a cold, but it didn't get better and it didn't go away. Within six weeks my lungs began to be affected. I had never suffered from asthma before, but I became asthmatic. I had episodes of coughing that would last for three hours at a time. These episodes became so severe I wound up with broken ribs as a result of all the hard coughing. As my illness progressed, I began to have terrible stomach problems, which led to constant vomiting. Between the coughing and the vomiting, I thought I was going to die. I developed incontinence. As if that wasn't enough, I also developed endometriosis."

Judith endured her illness for more than three years. During that time she was forced to leave her position at the hospital. "There was no way I could continue to do my job," she explained. "I was forced to take a breathing machine and adrenaline with me everywhere I went. Even if I could possibly gather the energy to work, nobody in a health facility would want to counsel with someone who was so awfully sick. Why would anyone trust me to help them when I had such awful problems myself? I was so incapacitated I pretty much became a recluse. I was confined to my house. The only time I left the house was to go to the doctor's office. I didn't have the strength to visit with any of my friends. My physical problems were not only constant, they were terribly embarrassing. They made it uncomfortable for me to even be around my own relatives. Still, I have to admit that develop-ing multiple chemical sensitivity was a wake-up call for me. When something like that happens, you find out who really cares about you. You find out who your friends are. I learned what was really important in life."

Even though Judith didn't know exactly what was causing her health to deteriorate, the one thing she did know was that she could not abandon hope. She could not give up her search for help. "I had so many things wrong with me that once they heard me tell them about all my different symptoms, the doctors gave up on me. I could see it in their eyes." She explained, "One time, after I had undergone a series of tests that came back from the lab with peculiar results, the doctor offered no advice. All he told me was: 'Beware of the ecolo-gists.' Then he walked out of the room. 'Beware of the ecologists.' I took it as a challenge."

Although that was not particularly helpful as a diagnosis, at least it gave her a clue to what might be causing her troubles. She continued to do research and to seek help. He research eventually led her to an environmental physician. "As soon as I got to him, I knew he was different," she said. "When you ask him a question, he'll give you a direct answer. He didn't give me any pat answers, and he didn't offer me any miracle cures. What he did was to teach me that I had to take responsibility for controlling my own illness. We talked a long time about my life, my work, and my surroundings. Then we did a series of tests. After that, he finally was able to make a diagnosis. After all that time I finally knew what was wrong with me."

Her program of detoxification was a revelation to her. She learned to consider issues in her personal environment that she would previously never have considered. She learned how to create a safe environment for herself in her own home. "I was really too sick to endure most of the testing. You might say I was too sick to find out how sick I really was. I had become so sensitive, I wasn't even able to take the allergy stuff, and I couldn't take the sauna treatments."

Judith's condition was helped dramatically when she began to take vitamin and mineral supplements. She learned how to avoid possible incitants. She believes that one of the most helpful aspects of her treatment was the opportunity to visit with other people who were suffering from the same disease.

"You sit there in the waiting room, or in the lab, or while you're waiting for your treatments, or even while you're taking your treatments, and you can't help but become friendly with the other patients. You're all in the same boat," she said. "Nobody else understands what you are going through in quite the way those other people understand. Other people tell you what they've got, and you tell them what you've got. These people know exactly what's wrong with you. They care about your symptoms, and they want to know what you have been doing to relieve them. They've walked in your shoes. They begin to become something like an extended family."

Judith insisted that the camaraderie she experienced was not simply a case of misery loves company. It offered the opportunity to exchange experiences, to share ideas about methods of coping with the sickness, and to speak with people who had survived, who were surviving, and who were returning to fairly normal lifestyles. "My doctor taught me about the environment," she said. "And the people I met during my treatments taught me that even though my life might not be exactly what it had been before, it was worth living. For the first time since I got sick I began to believe I really was going to live. You learn to take your sickness one day at a time, one week at a time, one year at a time. I heard several people saying they had been doing this for ten years, fifteen years, and more."

Her own situation became clear to her. "In searching for specific incitants, I realized I was reacting badly to just about everything around me. I came home and cleaned up my house and my surroundings. I learned exactly what caused me to have reactions, what I had to avoid, and how I could avoid these things. I eventually found my way to Dr. Edelson. He turned my life around."

Since beginning her recent course of treatments, Judith's life has improved dramatically. Although she still suffers from significant breathing problems, she is no longer obliged to carry a breathing machine with her wherever she goes. As a surprisingly positive result of her detoxification program, her endometriosis has entirely disappeared. She is careful to avoid specific incitants but she is no longer living the life of a recluse. She is no longer confined inside her house, too ashamed and embarrassed to be with other people. She considers multiple chemical sensitivity a wake-up call, both to those who suffer from it and to the rest of the world around her.

Although Judith is still unable to return to her former line of work, she has been able to use her degree and her experience in counseling to become an Alternative Health Consultant. She is determined to help other people achieve satisfactory levels of health. The most significant piece of advice she would offer to anyone who is suffering from multiple chemical sensitivity is this: "You can't listen to what the first person tells you. You can't listen to what the second person or even the third person tells you. You've got to continue to believe there's a way for you to return to health. You can't give up. You've got to keep trying until you find a doctor who will help you develop a life you can really live with."

8

Multiple Chemical Sensitivity Checklist

YOU PROBABLY have a good reason to think you are suffering from some environmentally related process if you have recently had a severe chemical exposure, find that you are sick and getting sicker, and that none of the steps you take, none of the medications you consume, nothing you do to improve your condition seems to help you to recover. Or perhaps you have been involved with work or with activities that constantly expose you to low levels of harmful chemicals and you discover that you have developed constant, unexplainable symptoms that will not go away. Could it be a single high-level exposure to a specific chemical that is making you ill? Or is it long-term exposure to low levels of a single specific chemical or a number of different chemicals? Perhaps you are a member of one of the groups identified as being at risk for chemical sensitivity?

Multiple chemical sensitivity affects many body functions important to the health of its victims. People suffering from multiple chemical sensitivity often become partially or totally disabled for several years or even for life. The stress associated with their conditions can lead to the disintegration of relationships. Sometimes they are forced to leave jobs they've held for some time or to leave high-level positions and deal with the devastating loss of income that results. However, with proper guidance and determination, there is hope that many people, even those with the most severe problems, can improve enough to return to work and to lead relatively normal lives.

It's also important to remember that the human mind and body are connected parts of a whole person. In addition to serious physical problems, chemical exposure can result in depression, erratic behavior, difficulty in concentrating, confusion, anxiety, peculiar body sensations, and headaches. Although the brain can be the target organ in some chemically sensitive people, its involvement should never be confused with psychosomatic disease. If nothing else, it is emotionally draining to know that your body can rebel against you at any time, at any place, during any activity, and that its symptoms may be stimulated by unusual odors, by perfumes, or by chemicals that don't seem to bother other people. You begin to have a hard time trusting your own body to be dependable in unusual situations. Eventually you may have a hard time trusting your own body to be dependable in the most normal, mundane situations.

But despite the diversity of symptoms the disorder can involve, doctors who have done research and have treated patients suffering from it usually agree on six diagnostic characteristics of multiple chemical sensitivity.

1. There is a variety of different symptoms involving a variety of different body systems such as the nervous system, the respiratory system, the gastrointestinal system, and the musculo-skeletal system.

2. Symptoms begin either after a particular exposure that can usually be identified by the person or after repeated low-level exposures.

3. Reactions are triggered by an increasing number of substances and products at lower and lower levels of exposure.

4. Symptoms can be brought on by very low levels of exposure, even those below the permissible exposure levels for various chemicals established by the United States government and usually below exposure levels generally acknowledged to be tolerated by most people.

5. Symptoms are triggered by exposures to a wide range of substances. These may include solvents in paint, varnishes, and adhesives. Pesticides and cleaning solutions are the most frequently recognized as triggering responses. Other substances can include such things as new building materials and new furniture, formaldehyde and the dyes used in manufacturing cloth and clothing, perfumes and colognes, detergents, car exhaust, books and newspapers, and copying machine and laser print toner.

6. No alternative explanations for the symptoms can be found.

If you think you are suffering from multiple chemical sensitivity, you may experience any number of debilitating ailments. Do you have severe, recurrent headaches or respiratory difficulties, asthma, joint pain, arthritis, depression, or symptoms of severe, debilitating and chronic fatigue that simply will not go away? Although you are constantly suffering, your symptoms might not always be constant and often depend on reactions to incitants to occur.

Have you visited your family doctor or several different doctors in your search for relief from your symptoms? Have you seen one or more specialists and consultants who attempted to treat your individual problems but were not able to explain the cause of your symptoms? Although you continue to take medications to alleviate your symptoms or to stop your pain, do the medications you are taking only seem to make your situation worse? No matter what you do, no matter how much medicine you take, no matter how many doctors you visit, you simply don't feel well. You are not yourself. You experience emotional problems, uncontrollable ups and downs, frustrating confusion, loss of memory, and difficulty in concentrating.

You may start to have so many symptoms of so many different diseases that your friends, your family, your coworkers, and even the medical professionals you visit in your search for help begin to doubt you. There are too many things wrong with you. You are simply too sick to be easily believed. At this point, everyone, even medical professionals, generally begin to label you a hypochondriac. You might even start to believe it yourself.

You know you have a problem when you find yourself going from doctor to doctor and experiencing a great deal of expensive, stressful, and even painful testing that finds nothing concrete to explain your many symptoms. Since they can't find out what's wrong with you, they send you to see a psychologist or a psychiatrist. Frustrated by the inability to pinpoint your illnesses, these professionals tell you that your symptoms are not real, that they are all in your head, and they stop listening to what you have to say about your problems.

But you know you are not making these symptoms up. They are very real and they are very painful. You know that you are not a malingerer. You don't have the time and you don't have the energy to be so sick, and you certainly aren't getting any pleasure out of it.

You may be suffering from multiple chemical sensitivity if you find that you have any or many of the following complaints. If you think your problem may be multiple chemical sensitivity, make your way to an environmental physician at once.

MCS Symptoms

- Adult onset acne
- Alopecia (sudden hair loss)
- Anxiety
- Arthritis
- Asthma
- Autoimmune diseases
- Central nervous system problems
- Chronic abdominal discomfort
- Chronic allergic illness
- Chronic ear infections
- Chronic fatigue syndrome
- Chronic neurological illness
- Chronic recurrent inflammation
- Chronic recurring infections
- Colitis
- Confusion
- Constant and incessant fatigue
- Crohn's disease
- Cystitis
- Depression
- Disorientation
- Dizziness
- Eczema
- Fainting spells
- Flulike symptoms

- Gastrointestinal problems
- Gynecological problems
- Headaches of all types
- Hyperactivity
- Increased sensitivity to certain odors
- Insomnia
- Irregular or rapid heartbeat
- Irritable bowel syndrome
- Irritability
- Joint pain
- Migraine headaches
- Multiple sclerosis
- Muscle pain
- Nasal problems, such as dryness
- Nausea
- Panic attacks
- PMS
- Psoriasis
- Rashes
- Redness and flushing
- Respiratory problems, such as asthma or other breathing problems
- Shortness of breath
- Short-term memory loss
- Skin disorders
- Spontaneous bruising

- Stuffy nose or chronic dry nose
- Swelling (edema)
- Tinnitus
- Unexplained fevers
- Vasculitis
- Vision problems
- Vulvodynia
- Weakness
- Yeast disease
- Yellowness of the skin without jaundice

9

Bill's Story

BILL EXPERIENCED EXPOSURE to all kinds of pesticides during the ten years he worked in the pest control business, but he didn't really get into trouble until he went into business for himself.

"It's true that when some people work with pesticides and other dangerous things over a long period of time they can develop a tendency to get careless," he admitted. "But that wasn't my problem. I knew how dangerous pesticides could be. My problem wasn't that I got careless. My problem was that I was trying to be too careful. When I went into business for myself, I bought only the finest and the best."

When he started his own pest control company he bought only first-rate equipment. "I got the best of everything," he said. "I bought all new equipment. Everything had to be top of the line. Since I had been working in the pest control business for such a long time, I knew what problems could be out there. At least I thought I knew. I didn't want anything that would cause any kind of problems. The trouble was that when you work in a business for a long time, you tend to get complacent. No matter how dangerous your products can be, when you work with them every day, they start to become so familiar that you forget about the dangers. Since I hadn't developed any problems I could recognize, and since I had bought the best equipment on the market, I didn't bother to wear any protective gloves for about a year and a half. Although I didn't know it, there was a small leak in my pesticide gun handle. It wasn't a big leak. It wasn't even anything you would notice. Small as that leak was, the pesticides were going directly into my system."

The first thing Bill noticed was an itch. Then he developed severe swelling of his extremities. "I was so swollen that all my veins disappeared in my body," he said. "I'd get hot working on a job and I'd go up on the mountain to cool off. Then, when I'd get into the cold air, I would become red and burning all over. I had night sweats."

Since his condition affected the nervous system, Bill suddenly had a tremendous amount of energy. "I'm a fairly energetic person to begin with, but I became terribly hyperactive. I was amazingly hyper, extremely hyper, unbearably hyper. I was an absolute nervous wreck. During that year and a half I was being pickled in chemicals right through the gun handle on my tank. I was getting this chemical exposure direct all week, every week, every day, for eight or ten hours at a time."

Bill also suffered from various other symptoms, but he was not aware that his other problems might be related to the chemicals he was using. "It affects your chest, and you don't even realize that you have a 'heavy' chest. The nerve endings are attached to your muscles, so that you feel as though you have a tremendous weight sitting right there on your chest. It happens so slowly and so subtly that you don't even realize what's going on. You don't know what's happening to you. I didn't realize I was being poisoned until much later."

His problems continued to get worse. "When I finally decided my problems had to be related to the chemicals I was using, it became obvious to me that it had to have something to do with the organic phosphate pesticide. It turned out I was right because when I finally found my way to help, they detected it."

When Bill realized that the poisons he was using against insects could be working against him, he decided to try wearing gloves at work. Shortly after he began using his gloves again, he noticed his symptoms became slightly less severe. "My hands had been covered with pure red spots. Because of the nerve endings, the tips of my fingers were covered with lines. It's hard to describe these markings. There were marks all the way down between the nail and the ends of my fingers. I didn't know exactly what caused it, but my nervous system was going crazy." Since the gloves seemed to help ease his symptoms, he wore two pair of neoprene gloves while he was working. "If you look carefully, you'll almost never see exterminators wearing neoprene gloves. That's because they cost at least $2.50 a pair," he explained. "Usually the exterminators will buy the cheapest things they can find. They'll buy cheap cotton gloves they can discard after they've been used a few times. I didn't want to do that. I knew I was being poisoned, and I didn't want to take any chances on letting that poison get through. It may be expensive, but neoprene is the best. It's the safest."

Bill made an appointment to see a dermatologist who prescribed an antihistamine to help relieve the unbearable itching he experienced. Although the antihistamine helped relieve the itch, it didn't do anything to improve any of his other symptoms. He kept visiting more doctors who prescribed more and more antihistamines.

"The truth was they didn't know what to do with me," he said. "Either they'd tell me, 'Something's really wrong with you,' or else they'd tell me, 'Nothing's really wrong with you. It's all in your mind.' By this time I had figured out that something was really wrong with me, and I also knew it wasn't only in my head. My mind wasn't making this one up. I was physically ill, and I knew there had to be a physical cause for it. In spite of all the drugs I was taking I wasn't getting any better."

Bill made an appointment with the lead doctor in the toxicology department at a major medical school in his area. "After they examined me, he and his assistant took urine specimens," he said. "That's all they did. They didn't do any blood chemistry work, nothing like that. The only thing they found out from their limited testing was that my body was high in zinc. I could have told them that. I knew I was high in zinc because I had been taking zinc tablets. I could see that they were completely baffled. Since they weren't able to find anything else that was wrong with me, they told me they couldn't do anything to help me. That wasn't too unreasonable. However, since they couldn't help me, they told me that nobody else could help me either. That was it. They told me there was no help for me."

By this time Bill's body was so swollen and he was so stressed he felt that he was ready to explode. "You talk about stressed out, burned-out, discouraged, disheartened, disappointed, and everything else," he remembered. "This thing affects your whole system and makes you unbearably sensitive. I'd become extremely sensitive to the light. All my skin was so sensitive that I developed dermatitis on my face. I started wearing a big hat and putting sunscreen all over me. My face finally cleared up, but it was still painful. I didn't know it at the time, but all this was going on because my immune system was broken down so badly. What I did know was that something was going to give. I believed that either I was going to have a heart attack or a stroke or something. There was just too much stress."

Discouraged, Bill began to believe there was no hope for improvement until an acquaintance recommended that he travel to Atlanta to see Dr. Edelson. "My wife and I were planning to take a trip to Maine," he said. "I decided that going to see this environmental doctor was a good idea. I told my wife, 'We'll be on the East Coast anyhow. What have we got to lose? Let's just drive down from Maine to Atlanta.'"

So they made their way to Atlanta. "When I walked into Dr. Edelson's office I felt as though a load was lifted from me," Bill said. "Somehow I knew I was going to get better. That man saved my life. If it wasn't for him I don't think I would have been here too much longer. People are slow to understand and learn new things, even if the things they're slow to learn and understand really do work. People often don't want to accept new ideas. They're hesitant, reluctant to change." He remarked, "I believe this type of molecular medicine is the medicine of the future. In the next twenty years they're going to discover that it truly works."

Bill spent six months in treatment, during which time he began to see marked improvement in his condition. In addition to Bill's other problems, Dr. Edelson diagnosed more than thirty food allergies.

"I remembered that I had some food allergies when I was a child growing up, but I thought I had outgrown them. I didn't know I still had any allergies. I just thought I had mucous coming up all the time. My eyes were always running. This tearing of the eyes is a symptom of organic phosphate poisoning, but it was also a symptom of my food allergies. After I had been poisoned, it became worse and worse."

During the first six months of his treatment Bill would return to Atlanta on and off for periods of five or six weeks at a time. "I've had about ninety IVs," he said. "I'm still not well but I'm a new person compared to where I was. Traveling back and forth from where I live to Atlanta is not a chore for me because I know how much it's going to help me. When the time comes, I'm ready to go back and get more treatment. I look forward to it!"

Even though his business was successful, Bill knew that his health would not allow him to continue working in pest control. "I'm a whole lot more fortunate than a lot of people who might have come down with this ailment," he said. "As I began to recover and to feel better, it became clear to me that I could not continue doing what I was doing. I had not planned to retire until I was much older, but since I owned my own business I was able to retire at the age of forty-eight. I can live comfortably now, but what's a whole lot more important is that I can look forward to living."

10

Sick Building Syndrome

SALLY IS A SINGLE MOTHER with the responsibility of raising three sons on her own. Under those difficult circumstances, she felt extremely fortunate to be able to work at a job she loved. Her work was varied and interesting, the people she worked with were congenial, the pay was good, and her employers were always appreciative of her capable intelligence and quiet charm.

Favored with employers and employees who all worked together toward a common goal, the company grew by leaps and bounds. It was so successful, it advanced and expanded until it had completely outgrown its original quarters. The decision was made to move from the old, less expensive, crowded, and somewhat time-worn surroundings into a brand new, energy-efficient high-rise office building.

"Our old place wasn't bad at all. In fact, it was really rather nice, but since we were growing so quickly and we were so busy, it had become overcrowded. There were so many desks and filing cabinets crowded together, there was hardly room for anyone to turn around.

The building we moved into was so new the paint was barely dry on the walls. The new offices were absolutely beautiful," Sally said. "They were plush. They had softly painted walls and wonderful lighting. They had every convenience we could possibly have dreamed about."

Unfortunately, moving into the beautiful new headquarters marked the beginning of Sally's problems. "I sneezed my way through the move," she said, "then coughed and sneezed my way through the first few weeks after the move. I suddenly began to develop allergies I'd never had before. I became sensitive to all sorts of pollens, dust, foods, mold, and dampness. I was tired all the time, but I had been working so hard during the move I figured that was to be expected. I didn't think too much about it. I thought that being so tired was a natural result of the move combined with the stress and the change of surroundings."

When her health and exhaustion did not improve, Sally suspected her problems were made worse because the designer had placed her desk directly under an air conditioning outlet. She had the location of her desk changed, but the change didn't help. She continued to become sicker and sicker. Her normally dynamic energy level decreased until it had completely failed. She would drag herself home from work at the end of the week on Friday, rest during the weekend, and return to work on Monday only to suffer from renewed exhaustion and rapidly deteriorating respiratory problems. Only one other employee on the company's staff developed similar problems. Since both women were approximately the same age, Sally's family doctor suggested they were both experiencing menopausal difficulties. "I had heard all the old wives' tales about how menopause brought many women serious physical and emotional difficulties, but I'd never heard anybody say that bronchitis was one of them," Sally laughed. "As my health continued to get worse, I started to look for another explanation. Why would I begin to feel a little better on the weekends only to get sick again when I went back to work?"

Her friends suggested there was a psychosomatic cause. Perhaps the real problem was her job. Some of her friends hinted that she secretly hated her job but she dared not admit it, not even to herself. Some of her friends even suggested she see a psychiatrist.

"The only trouble with that idea was that I didn't hate my job at all. I liked everybody and I liked everything about it except the new office building with its sealed up windows and sealed up doors. Nothing could get into that building. Those sealed up windows were tinted brown so that not even the sun could come in." It wasn't what couldn't come in to the new building that was causing Sally's problems. Although she didn't know it at the time, her suffering was caused by the pollution that couldn't get out.

"I know it's strange for a sensible person to hate an inanimate object, but I began to hate that big shiny new office building," she explained. "As irrational as it seemed to me at the time, I felt as though that building had become an oppressive presence in my life. When I was at home all weekend and I would start to feel a little better, I would be able to function in a normal way. Then Monday would come around and I would have to go back to work in that awful building. After I had been there for a few hours, I would get sick all over again. By the end of the week, I could barely haul myself home from work. I knew I couldn't go on like that, getting sicker and sicker. I was pretty much alone in the world, and my kids had nobody to depend on but me. What would happen to them if I became seriously ill? I couldn't let that happen. I didn't know exactly what I had to do, but I knew I had to do something."

She heard about an opportunity to go to work for another company. Changing jobs not only involved a major cut in pay but the unhappy prospect of commuting to a nearby town as well. She would be leaving the job she enjoyed and the many friends she had made at work, but she knew she couldn't let the opportunity pass her by. She made the change.

In spite of having to leave the company she helped to build, in spite of losing her friends, losing money in the job change, and facing the long commute from one town to the next, Sally's story has a happy ending. Within days she felt her health begin to improve. She stopped her illness soon enough, her toxic load was limited enough, and her body's systems were strong enough to allow her to recover by simply removing herself from the sick building. The presence of fewer severe sneezing and coughing spells allowed her to recapture her cheerful outlook. Her bronchitis became less severe. Her energy slowly began to return.

She is still sensitive to pollens, dust, certain foods, molds, and dampness. She can't wear or even be near woolen clothing or perfumed products and is never quite sure when her respiratory problems will reappear, but she is convinced that making the job change helped her to rescue her health. "Even now some of my friends think the whole thing was psychological and my doctor still thinks it was menopausal," Sally said. "But I know it was that office building. I won't even go back into that place to visit my old friends. When they want to see me, they can meet me somewhere else."

We become so concerned with the pollution of the outside world that few, if any, of us ever stop to consider that our health might be assaulted by indoor air pollution. Our homes, factories, schools, shops, and offices were once equipped with windows that could be opened to vent unpleasant smells and to clear away the unfortunate effects of visible pollutants. But that has all changed.

During the acute energy crisis of the 1970s we actually paid high-priced consultants to show us where our expensively heated or cooled air was "leaking" out of our buildings. We bought gallons of caulking and ribbons of window sealer as we rushed to make our doors and windows weathertight and airtight. We hurried to plug the leaks and seal ourselves inside. Many schools and businesses actually nailed the windows shut, both to keep valuable heat and cool air inside and to cut down on vandalism and theft from outside.

On a national scale, our leaky old offices, hotels, hospitals, shops, schools, and homes gave way to new energy-efficient construction, much of it designed with windows that could never be opened, or worse, with no windows at all. We had no desire to bring unheated and uncooled outdoor air inside, nor did we want to allow any of our precious indoor air to get out.

As a result of this rush to preserve energy, ventilation requirements that demanded the introduction of outdoor air into commercial buildings were seriously reduced. Volatile chemicals began seeping into our carefully weatherproof, leakproof, energy-efficient buildings with their reduced ventilation requirements. And they started poisoning the people who lived and worked inside. At the same time, an array of new chemicals was introduced into the building trades, providing advanced methods of construction and economical, prefabricated decoration.

Indoor air can become contaminated by mixtures of toxic chemicals that come from new furniture, new carpets, and improved pesticides, as well as from stagnant or contaminated water allowed to remain in air conditioning systems. A dangerous situation is created when these problems are combined with inadequate building ventilation.

Environmental Protection Agency (EPA) researchers have recorded organic chemicals in air samples from countless indoor environments. Newly renovated buildings show higher than average chemical levels. The chemical toluene emanates from paints, and formaldehyde is released from new carpeting. But employees also introduce chemicals into indoor environments. Dry-cleaned fabrics contain chlorinated hydrocarbons and neurotoxic substances. Ingredients in cologne, aftershave, and perfume are intentionally designed to remain in the air for hours. Our beautiful new buildings are sick, and they are making us sick.

Sick building syndrome causes health problems like eye, nose, and throat irritation; sinus discomfort; headaches; sneezing; coughing; respiratory infections; fatigue; nausea; rashes; and dizziness. These symptoms are also common to multiple chemical sensitivity.

The majority of these symptoms will improve or even disappear in most people when they leave the building, when the building's ventilation is improved, or when the offending substance or substances are removed or replaced. But it is possible that sick building syndrome precedes multiple chemical sensitivity. For people whose total body load has been reached or surpassed, or for those who are genetically at risk to develop multiple chemical sensitivity, indoor air pollution may trigger its symptoms.

In addition to people who spend their days in large office buildings, school teachers have been identified as a major group of people who are significantly at risk for developing chemical problems. Classrooms are often painted, carpeted, and treated with air fresheners, pesticides, and powerful cleaning materials. They are filled with dust mites living in books, chalk dust, glues, paints, and other classroom materials. The newest school buildings have neither windows that open nor adequate ventilation.

Students as well as teachers can suffer from the effects of fungi and microbes in faulty air-conditioning and ventilation systems; from dust, mold, and pollen; and fumes from synthetic carpets and furnishings, building materials, and classroom supplies. However, students typically spend only one hour a day in offending classrooms while teachers remain in the same room eight hours a day, five days a week. Their bodies can become seriously compromised by the chemical overload.

The same may be true for a family that has moved into a new home or has remodeled an existing home. Family members who remain at home all day can suffer more intense chemical exposure from new building materials, carpeting, paints, glues, and dyes than those who work outside the home and only spend a few hours at home in the evening.

Sick Building Syndrome

The United States government issues standards for permissible exposure levels (PELs) to toxic chemicals. These minimum standards were developed for industrial workers who have frequent contact with hazardous chemicals. At least these people have the advantage of knowing they are at risk. These standards were not, however, developed for office workers, teachers, schoolchildren, and people who are living in the alleged comfort and safety of their own homes. There are no specific federal standards for the quality of indoor air in office buildings, schools or homes.

And unfortunately, even if government standards were applied to these areas, they would be inadequate to protect people who are chemically sensitive. Such people experience symptoms of illness after they are exposed to concentrations of chemicals that are far below the standards set for industry. Whole buildings can be affected by chemical exposure. When the national headquarters of the EPA in Washington DC was stricken with sick building problems, however, the situation became too embarrassing to be ignored.

The incident was reported by B. Hileman in "Multiple Chemical Sensitivity" (*Chemical Engineering News*, July 22, 1991). It seems that in 1988 new carpeting was installed in the EPA's office building. Ventilation rates in the EPA offices were particularly low to satisfy energy-efficiency standards of temperature control. Within days after the carpeting was installed, employees in the building began to complain about burning eyes, rashes, dizziness, respiratory problems, and nausea. Within months, 122 of the two thousand employees became sick. It turned out that the new carpeting was the villain. Employees' health problems were traced to unsatisfactory indoor air quality as well as to chemical emissions from the new carpeting. This led to the naming of the phenomenon "sick building syndrome," or "tight building syndrome."

Even though the offensive carpeting was removed, forty-five to fifty of the employees had been so severely sensitized by carpet fumes, combined with emissions from additional new building materials, that they were unable to return to the building without becoming ill. Reasonable accommodations were made so that these people were able to continue to work at home or in offices that had bare floors and were equipped with functioning windows.

And although most of the EPA's employees who were involved appear to have been able to rid the hazardous chemicals from their bodies, some of them may gradually develop symptoms of multiple chemical sensitivity over a period time. They may begin to react when they come into contact with chemicals such as perfumes and auto exhausts, which never bothered them before, or they may develop sensitivities to foods that never bothered them before.

People who suffer from multiple chemical sensitivity do have rights. Two major federal agencies, the Federal Housing and Urban Development (HUD) and the Social Security Administration, have recognized multiple chemical sensitivity as a disability. The Americans with Disabilities Act, which became law July 26, 1990, extends its protection to the estimated forty-three million disabled Americans and guarantees equal opportunity for people with such disabilities in employment, public accommodations, transportation, and other services. However, as with all other illnesses, recognition of multiple chemical sensitivity under the Americans with Disabilities Act is determined on a case-by-case basis.

Reasonable accommodations can involve simple modifications that can be made to a work environment that enables qualified people with disabilities to perform their jobs. They allow them to continue be productive, working members of society instead of being fired or forced to resign and becoming dependent upon disability insurance.

Reasonable accommodations can be made for chemically sensitive employees. Many such accommodations can be accomplished at little or no cost to the employer. Certain areas might be designated as smoke-free and fragrance-free working and eating areas. Affected employees may be allowed to avoid coming into contact with dry-cleaned fabrics, cologne, aftershave, and perfume ingredients that contain petrochemicals and neurotoxic substances. Another accommodation can be made by selecting the least toxic or allergenic building furniture and supplies. Affected employees can, and should, be notified in advance when building renovations, construction, painting, and pesticide applications are planned. Provisions can be made for alternative working arrangements until these changes are completed.

Such reasonable accommodations are cost effective because they can help employers to retain highly skilled, well-trained, and valued employees. However, employers are not required to provide reasonable accommodation if doing so imposes undue hardship, significant difficulty, or expense to the functioning of a business. Since indoor air pollution costs businesses an estimated one hundred billion dollars a year in lost work time, insurance, and health-care payments, it makes good business sense to address indoor air problems. It certainly is important for homes and schools to address such problems.

Indoor air quality can be improved by simple, efficient, and cost-effective means. Most of the time, such improvements can be made at little or no cost to the employer. Flexibility and creativity can go a long way.

Ten Ways to Improve Indoor Air Quality

1. Install windows that open or unblock windows that have been permanently closed or sealed.

2. Clean and maintain ventilation systems and open or unblock all additional sources of fresh air.

3. Adapt current ASHRAE (American Society of Heating, Refrigeration, and Air Conditioning Engineers) ventilation standards, which require twenty cubic feet per minute per

person of fresh air in an office or workplace. It is important to remember that ASHRAE standards are minimal and don't include special accommodations for the chemically sensitive.

4. Be sure that all local exhaust systems pull polluted air away from areas where people work.

5. Vent office machines such as photocopiers, laser printers, and computer terminals that release toxic chemicals.

6. Select the least toxic or nontoxic building furnishings and supplies.

7. Avoid the use of toxic chemicals. Substitute less dangerous materials. This is particularly important in cleaning, pest control, and renovation work.

8. Eliminate pesticide applications, painting with toxic paints, and renovations using toxic materials.

9. Contain smoking in special vented or outdoor smoking areas or prohibit it entirely by becoming a nonsmoking facility.

10. Install heat exchangers that recover heat or cooling while increasing fresh-air inflow. This provides more circulation and cuts energy costs.

Improving the quality of indoor air as an accommodation for the chemically sensitive improves air quality for everyone. We all benefit from a cleaner and safer environment.

11

Susie's Story

BRIGHT, ATTRACTIVE, and hard working, Susie always considered herself to be a healthy person. She never got sick. Friends and relatives admired Susie and her husband because they were so happy together, so young and so energetic. They had a wonderful life. Susie's coworkers nicknamed her "Little Susie Sunshine," for her outgoing personality and her cheerful, upbeat ways. Six months later, though, "Little Susie Sunshine" was desperately ill.

"The worst part was that I got sick at work," she said. "I truly enjoyed my job. I worked there for five years before this started, and I felt as though the people I worked with had become my family." Susie worked in the office of a small construction company. Workmen came into the office every morning. The company's owners parceled out the day's assignments, after which both the owners and the workmen went off to do their jobs. Susie was the only employee who remained in the building through the entire eight-hour workday.

One morning, a hurried workman carelessly placed a five-gallon container of concrete sealer on top of the insulation-wrapped heat duct in the furnace room, which was also used as a storeroom. Susie noticed the strong odor as soon as she entered the building later that morning. Since the odor reminded her of paint fumes, she asked her employer if they had been painting the building, but he told her they had not. Although her employer had also noticed the odor, the only suggestion he could offer was that the odor might be the result of fumes coming from the cars and trucks parked in the building's attached garage.

Since it was unpleasant enough to be disruptive, Susie and her employer began to look for the source of the odor. Before they could find it, however, he was called away to a construction job. When his partner arrived, he also joined Susie in looking for the source of the odor, but again they were unable to locate it. He was also called away to a job. He suggested that Susie open the building's doors and leave them open. Perhaps the mysterious odor would simply go away.

"I opened the doors for a little while, but I knew I had to shut them. Of course you can't keep the doors to a business office wide open all day. This was a business office, after all, and it didn't look businesslike," Susie said. "It was necessary to keep up professional appearances. Besides, it was summer, and it was hot outside. With the doors open and all that hot air coming in from outside, the air conditioner was forced to run at top speed."

Susie closed the doors, recirculating the air through the building. After all she thought, it was only a smell.

The bottom of the five-gallon plastic container had not been sealed properly, so the concrete sealer had leaked into the heating and air conditioning duct. The dangerous liquid continued to seep into the office air supply for nine full months.

"I was so sick by lunchtime that first day I could hardly stand it," Susie said. "I had a headache and irritated sinuses. I felt as though I was coming down with an attack of hay fever, although it wasn't hay fever season. By supper time I was suffering with nausea and diarrhea. I decided it couldn't be hay fever. I thought I had somehow come down with the flu. By the end of the week I was so sick I don't know how I functioned, if I functioned, or when I functioned at all. I was dizzy all the time. I was so dizzy I don't know how I dared to get behind the wheel to drive my car. Still, I went to work every day, even when I was so sick I could barely stand."

When she answered the telephone, the firm's regular customers, who were familiar with her voice, told Susie she sounded as though she had a cold. She knew she didn't have a cold because a cold would have gone away, and her respiratory problems continued to linger on and on. "I didn't know exactly what I had," she said. "But I knew I didn't have anything contagious. Since I knew I couldn't infect anyone else, I kept dragging myself to work and doing the best I could."

Worse than the respiratory difficulties, Susie experienced changes in her vision. These changes were followed by extreme depression. She started to gain weight. Her self-esteem plummeted. In a vain effort to lose the excess weight she had gained, she began to eat less and less food. The more she starved herself, the more weight she gained. She tried every kind of weight-loss diet she could find—crash diets, health-food diets, and even sensible diets. Nothing she could do seemed to help her to lose weight. She developed painfully dry skin. She began to notice huge black circles forming around her eyes. She tried to rest as much as possible to overcome her constant exhaustion. But regardless of how much rest she got, she remained tired all the time.

"We live a block away from a main road," she said. "Workmen doing road repairs dug up the asphalt. The dust from those road repairs made me unbearably sick. I had asked our apartment manager not to spray for insects, but I was gone one day and the exterminator came into our apartment and sprayed in spite of my request. The insect spray triggered a violent reaction. I was sick for days."

Once Susie tripped and fell down the stairs. Bruises that normally would have healed in a short time took more than three months to heal. As a result of the fall, she wound up with shingles. "The chemicals I was exposed to affected my immune system and shut it down," she explained. "My immune system had become so compromised that nothing worked the way it should."

She also found herself having difficulty concentrating. Her normal typing speed of sixty-five or seventy words a minute slowed to forty words a minute or less. Worse, she started to make errors in the company's bookkeeping and in the payroll.

As the multiple chemical sensitivity compromised her body's physical systems, it also effected her emotional well-being. "I cried all the time," she said. "I could barely do anything that didn't make me cry. I would get up in the morning, haul myself to work, sit at my desk trying to concentrate on my job, and I would start to cry."

She was also unable to sleep at nights. She would sleep for only an hour or two at most, then she would get up and walk around the house, terrified that someone was attempting to break in. "I became extremely paranoid," she said. "I decided the locks we had on the doors were not strong enough to protect me." She demanded more and more locks, more bars, more chains.

"My family was beside themselves worrying and wondering what was happening to me. They couldn't imagine that someone who was sick would develop the kinds of terrible fears I had. They couldn't imagine that someone who was sick would have some of the peculiarities I began to develop," she remembered. "I wouldn't even talk to my closest friends. When my friends called to talk to me, my husband would have to tell them, 'I'm sorry, but Susie can't come to the phone right now.' And it was the truth. I really couldn't come to the phone. I really couldn't talk. My friends didn't understand. They had no way to understand. Even my husband didn't understand."

The illness also caused problems in Susie's marriage. "I adore my husband. Ours is a marriage built on love and trust, but at one point I decided my husband was having an affair with a woman who worked at his office. The harder he denied it the stronger I believed it. One day I got so upset I started smashing plates and dishes. I was just throwing things and screaming. I told him I was leaving him. He couldn't calm me. I was hysterical. It was unreal."

Although her life seemed to be falling apart, Susie continued to do her work as best she could. Nine months after that first massive chemical exposure, she finally found out what she had been breathing all that time. "It was the last day of October and the weather had started to turn cold. It was really chilly in the office so we decided to turn on the heat. When we turned on the heating unit the smell in the office magnified. I was convinced that whatever was causing that smell had to be coming from the furnace storeroom. I asked one of the workmen to help me clean out the storeroom. He started to carry out all the big heavy things. When he picked up the five-gallon container of concrete sealer and set it in the hallway, it left a huge wet spot on the carpet. We went back into the storeroom and found a depressed area on the insulation where the container had been sitting all those months. The insulation was saturated with that stuff. The floor was saturated. They could have blown up the building by simply lighting a match."

After Susie read the container's label she began to look through the files for product safety information. She found none. When you buy a product like that they don't give you that kind of information," she explained. "Nobody tells us how hazardous such products can be. We all tend to think that just because we can buy something in a store, it's safe for us to use."

Susie called the manufacturer and received an eight-page product-safety sheet. Manufacturers are obliged by law to provide product safety sheets that disclose all the contents and potential hazards. She discovered that that particular concrete sealer was carcinogenic, and it was also known to cause a variety of other serious health problems.

Her employers advised her to see a doctor. She had already seen her general practitioner. He had been treating her sinus infections with antibiotics, which only seemed to make her situation worse. After her doctor read the product-safety sheet and saw a list of all her symptoms, he referred her to a pulmonary specialist.

Ailing, exhausted, frightened, and unable to concentrate, Susie felt that she was living a nightmare. However, her medical nightmare had only begun. "They put me on a merry-go-round, going from doctor to doctor to doctor," she said. "All of them insisted on giving me different tests. Those test were not only painful, they were expensive. After we had completed a series of medical tests, they would say, 'Yes, you have some respiratory problems' or 'Yes, you have bronchitis.' It was nice of them to tell me that, but I already knew it. I didn't need them to tell me I was sick. What I needed was for them to tell me how I could get well.

But Susie didn't get well. "I kept getting sicker. That made me meaner and more nervous until each of the doctors would give up on me and send me off to see somebody else. When they couldn't figure out what was wrong with me, they started to send me to psychiatrists. I even went to a toxicologist who did some blood tests and some motor-function tests. When he couldn't find anything wrong with me, he also decided I should go see a psychiatrist.

"I saw a psychiatrist and a psychologist who both told me I had decreased motor function and short-term memory problems. Before it was all over I wound up going to three different psychiatrists and three different psychologists. They all told me I was moderately to severely depressed and suicidal. I had never once thought about death or dying until they told me I was suicidal. I said, 'I don't want to die. I want to live. I want to be well. I want to be my old self again.' "

Susie was angry with everybody and everything. "I was particularly angry at the way the insurance company treated me," she said. My employers knew that I did indeed get sick at work. I worked for them for five years before this happened. They knew the sort of person I was. They knew I wasn't trying to get something I didn't deserve."

Susie innocently sent her medical bills to the Workman's Compensation carrier. They promptly refused her expenses. "We don't believe you got sick at work," they told her. "Why would you be the only one to get sick when nobody else got sick?"

After they refused her medical expenses, she had no choice but to seek help from an attorney. "The first thing the attorney asked me was, 'Do you ever want to get well?' I said, 'Of course I do.'

"Then he asked, 'If you really want to get well, why do you continue to go in there every day and resaturate your body with all those chemicals? That's where your sickness is coming from. It's in the walls, it's in the furniture. It's in everything your breathe and touch. If you want to get well you cannot go back to work there.'"

Susie had seen the attorney on Friday. The following Monday she was obliged to tell her employers she was leaving. She couldn't work for them anymore. Leaving her job was almost as hard for her to endure as being sick.

"I left the job I loved and the people I loved and went to a world of battling my way from this doctor to the next doctor, of battling with the insurance company, of battling with the insurance company's attorneys," she remembered. "The sickness was bad enough, but the legal part of it was horrible to deal with. They made me feel as though I was some kind of common criminal, as though I had done something wrong to bring this on myself. I was suffering physical and mental pain, and their attorneys were asking me questions about my past, about how much money my husband earned, about all sorts of things that had no bearing on my situation."

The attorney for the insurance company suffered from chemical sensitivity himself. "He knew exactly what I was going through," Susie said. "He knew exactly how bad off I was, but he also had the job of representing his insurance company. By this time I even became depressed about the way my attorney was handling my case. Following my attorney's advice, we settled our case the day before we went to court. After we had settled, the attorney for the insurance company told my attorney, 'I was convinced she would win the case if we ever went into court.' But we didn't go to court. It turns out we had a very conservative judge presiding, so my attorney felt it would be better to settle the case than to take chances on an unpredictable court trial. He settled by accepting less than half the amount we knew was necessary to cover my medical treatments. The treatment I wanted to have would have cost twenty-five thousand dollars. I already had fifty thousand dollars worth of medical expenses to pay, and there was no way I could afford the additional treatment even though I believed it might have helped me to improve. Since I couldn't afford it, I was determined to go from day to day doing the best I could."

Surprisingly, it turned out to be Susie's attorney who eventually found the appropriate medical help for her. "It was one of those almost impossible, unbelievable chance happenings," she explained. "My attorney was invited to a party where he found himself talking with another attorney who represented a woman in Atlanta who had suffered from a severe chemical reaction to insect spray. As they spoke he realized that her symptoms were very much like my symptoms. With her permission, the attorneys got the two of us together by phone. The woman told me about her problems. It was somehow comforting to me to find someone who had similar problems to mine. She encouraged me and told me there was help for me. She gave me Dr. Edelson's name and phone number.

"When I first went to see Dr. Edelson, I took a notebook with me, and because that wasn't enough, I also took my husband with me. My short-term memory had been so badly compromised I was certain I wouldn't be able to remember anything the doctor might tell me. I was amazed when he listened to what I had to say without judging me or acting as though he thought I was crazy. He understood everything

I was talking about. It was easy for me to see he'd heard it all before. I would describe my symptoms to him, and he would give me additional information. He said we needed to do some testing to see exactly what was happening to me physically, and then we would do some other testing to see what was happening to me emotionally. Although it meant even more testing, I didn't complain. I somehow knew that here was someone who was going to find a way to help me."

Susie spent most of the next month at the doctor's office. "There were basically no drugs, no antibiotics. I went on a liquid rice diet for three weeks so that I could clean out my body. Then I started taking different types of nutritional supplements to help build my immune system back up to help fight off viral or bacterial infections. During that time, I cleaned all the chemical products out of my house. We've been partners in working with my problems. Together, we've treated my illness by avoiding things that cause me to have reactions You never really know what incitant is going to harm you. You never really know where this sickness is going to hit you next."

It has been necessary for Susie and her husband to make certain extreme lifestyle changes. She can't wear make up. She must avoid all perfumed products. "That is really difficult to do," she said. "Virtually all the popular consumer products we use in our homes today are scented in one form or another."

She must avoid dish detergent, laundry detergent, fabric softeners, bar soap, room deodorants, air fresheners, hair spray, and the people who routinely use these products. "At first it was hard for my husband to avoid using all those products, and it was hard for people who wanted to come and visit us because I'd have to say, 'Please don't wear your normal perfume or aftershave lotion when you come to see me.' People from our church wanted to visit me. They're good people, and their feelings were hurt when they came to our door and we wouldn't let them come in. If they were wearing perfumed products, we couldn't let them in. They understood I was sick, but they didn't understand why a sick person couldn't be in the same room with someone who was wearing aftershave lotion."

Susie even had to stop reading the morning newspaper because she suffered from reactions to the ink used in the newsprint. It triggered breathing difficulties. She also had to stop reading her favorite magazines because of reactions to the perfumed inserts.

Some of the lifestyle changes she had to make were extremely difficult. Susie had enjoyed creative art. She had even participated in a crafts co-op. She can never do that again. Still, she insisted that as difficult as these changes may have been, she embraced them because it was such a relief for her not to suffer from reactions to chemical substances.

With all of this, Susie has developed a greater appreciation for life. "I used to think I would live forever. I was so happy and healthy, and everything in my life was so positive and perfect. Since I've been sick I've learned there are more important things in life than having a job. There are more important things than having money. I've been able to help other people make changes in their lives. It would make me extremely happy if I could prevent this nightmare from happening to someone else."

Even so, she can't help but wonder what would her life would have been like if she had been more outspoken during the first week of her exposure. "What would have happened if I had just said, 'That smell is making me sick. We've got to find out where it's coming from and get rid of it,' she wondered.

"With treatment and care I have been able to return to a reasonably normal lifestyle," she explained. "But I know that I will never be completely well. People like me, people who have so many chemical sensitivities don't dare kid ourselves. We have to face the truth. Even though I have responded well to my treatment and I have taken many positive steps forward, I always have to keep reminding myself to do this or to do that. I always have to be careful about where I go and what I do. I will always have to be aware of my surroundings. Still, as long as I can take all the necessary precautions, I feel as though I'm in control of my life again. I know I can stay as well as possible and not get worse. "

12

Understanding Your Rights

Two MAJOR federal agencies, HUD and the Social Security Administration, have recognized multiple chemical sensitivity as a disability. The Americans with Disabilities Act (ADA) of 1990 may also affect those with the disorder. The ADA extends protections to the estimated forty-three million disabled Americans and guarantees equal opportunity for people with disabilities in employment, public accommodations, transportation, and other services. The ADA defines a person with a disability as anyone with "a physical or mental impairment that substantially limits one or more of the major life activities, a record of such impairment, or being regarded as having such impairment."

ADA recognition of multiple chemical sensitivity is determined on a case-by-case basis, as with all other illnesses. The Justice Department will not state categorically that allergies or sensitivities are disabilities. However, the department does note that individuals with severe sensitivities that limit one or more major life activities may meet the ADA definition of disabled.

If you are disabled by multiple chemical sensitivity, you have the right, by law, to ask for reasonable accommodations in your workplace. An excellent guide to what reasonable accommodations are is a thirty-two-page booklet called "Reasonable Accommodation: A Guide for Employers, Businesses and Persons with Disabilities." It is published by the Governor's Committee on Disability Issues and Employment in Washington state and can be obtained by calling (206) 438-3168.

Basically, reasonable accommodation is a modification or adjustment made to a job or a work environment (including recruitment and training) that enables an otherwise qualified person with a disability to perform the job. Below are some examples of reasonable accommodation for a chemically sensitive worker.

- An office with a window that opens
- Designated smoke-free and fragrance-free work and eating areas
- Prenotification of building renovations, construction, painting, and pesticide applications with provisions for alternative work arrangements
- Selection of least toxic building furnishings and supplies
- Eliminating the use of air fresheners, deodorizers, potpourri, and disinfectants through the building, ventilation system, and individual automatic dispensers
- Allowing flextime, part-time work, or the option to work at home in order to avoid fully staffed offices, rush-hour traffic (exposure to automobile fumes), and crowded buses and subways (exposure to consumer products)
- Providing daylight or incandescent light rather than fluorescent lighting

- Providing errand runners for employees who may be affected by substances (perfumes, colognes, auto exhaust) normally encountered in the course of conducting office business

- Making provisions for closed-circuit televisions, interactive computers, and conference-call mechanisms that can be used either in a "safe" room in the office or from the individual's home

- Educating coworkers and supervisors about chemical sensitivity to promote positive attitudes and actions

- Removing carpets or selecting the least toxic flooring and adhesives

These are common examples of reasonable accommodation, but even further measures have been taken by some employers. In one case, the courts mandated one employer to protect nonsmokers. Two employees who worked for the County of Fresno in California were seriously affected by tobacco smoke. Their employer was instructed by the courts to institute reasonable accommodations. These included providing smokers with desktop air filtration machines, keeping windows open, separating smokers' desks from nonsmokers' desks, moving sensitive individuals to private offices, and allowing one employee to take an unpaid leave of absence.

In yet another instance, a union local won the right for a chemical-free exam site. CSEA Local 690 won the right for people with chemical sensitivities to take a Civil Service exam at an alternative location. Originally, the exam was scheduled to be given at a local high school known for frequent pesticide use.

By law, employers are not required to provide reasonable accommodation if such accommodations impose an undue hardship (a significant difficulty or expense) on the functioning of the business. However, it makes good business sense for an employer to work with an employee to develop a reasonable working situation. So, if you are chemically sensitive and plan to talk to your employer about making accommodations, here are some strong business points to make:

- Job accommodation doesn't need to be expensive. A little flexibility and creativity go a long way. Many accommodations involve no cost to the employer. It will probably cost an employer more money to hire and retrain a new employee than to accommodate an experienced one.

- An accommodation is probably less expensive in the long run than a court battle, which an employee has the option to pursue.

- Many of the accommodations made for an employee with multiple chemical sensitivity (like those affecting air quality) will benefit the entire staff by providing a cleaner and safer work environment that can prevent potential health problems and absenteeism.

What Is the Government Doing about MCS?

Unfortunately, not much. Only two states, Maine and New Hampshire, have legislation on indoor air quality. Their laws require that ventilation systems in all newly leased and constructed state and government buildings conform to ASHRAE standards. ASHRAE standards state that fresh outdoor air should be adequately distributed during the entire time office space is in use at a minimum rate of twenty cubic feet per minute per person. These laws, however, do not apply to the private sector.

California has an indoor air standard that requires that ventilation systems must be on at all times when a building is occupied. This standard affects custodial workers who often perform their jobs after normal business hours. The legislature is also considering a bill to require "bake outs" of all new public buildings, which would detoxify a build-ing (a seven-day process) to get rid of contaminants associated with new construction.

New Jersey has indoor air quality regulations for public employees. The rules set standards for indoor air legislation and provide a means for workers to make formal complaints about indoor air quality prob-lems. Key provisions include the following: renovation work must be isolated and ventilated; air from smoking areas may not be recircu-lated to nonsmoking areas; area managers must follow a maintenance schedule for HVAC systems.

Washington state is also establishing detailed minimum ventilation requirements for all buildings except residences and factories.

New York's Right-to-Know Law gives every worker the right to information about the substances they work with on the job. This law covers all chemicals, asbestos, radiation, and infectious diseases. Most of the information can be found in MSDSA or chemical fact sheets. According to this law employers must provide the following:

- Right-to-know signs or posters located in the workplace that include the name and telephone number of the person or agency to contact to obtain MSDSAs or other information about chemicals

- The names of the products used on the job as well as their manufacturers

- The chemical composition of the product

- The short- and long-term health effects

- The level of exposure that may be hazardous and the range of symptoms of exposure (headaches, dizziness, shortness of breath, etc.)

- Ways to reduce exposure: proper ventilation, respirators, skin and eye protection, etc.

- Fire, explosion, and reactivity information
- Emergency response to leaks, spills, and other accidents
- Emergency and first-aid instructions

Permissible Exposure Levels

The US government issues standards for permissible exposure levels (PELs) to toxic chemicals.

Unfortunately, government standards are inadequate to protect multiple chemical sensitivity sufferers. These minimum standards were developed for industrial workers who have frequent contact with hazardous chemicals. They were not developed for office workers, teachers, schoolchildren, and people living in the alleged safety of their own homes. Those who are chemically sensitive experience symptoms of illness after exposure to concentrations of chemicals that are far below the standards set for industry. And there simply are no federal standards for the quality of indoor air in office buildings or schools.

The first standards were set by the Occupational Safety and Health Administration (OSHA) in 1970. But standards for toxic substances were not issued until 1989, the same year OSHA developed standards for 428 toxic substances. These standards were based on the threshold limit values (TLVs), which were established by the American Conference of Governmental Industrial Hygienists. This nongovernmental group provided guidelines for government contractors based largely on information supplied to them by corporations.

The National Institute of Occupational Safety and Health (NIOSH), a government agency, recommended standards based on available scientific data. Many of NIOSH's recommendations are stricter than the PELs adopted by OSHA. For example, the *Pocket Guide to Chemical Hazards*, published by the NIOSH in June 1990, recommends a standard for arsenic that is two micrograms per cubic meter. OSHA's standard is ten micrograms. OSHA ignored the recommendations of NIOSH. So, even if a company observes OSHA standards, the health of its workers may still be in danger.

13

Rick's Story

RICK WAS A WORKAHOLIC. He would be the first to admit it. He loved his work almost to the point of obsession, working sixteen- to eighteen-hour days and enjoying every minute of it. He was a single young man, healthy, out on his own, working for a major computer corporation and so completely involved in what he was doing that he was neither eating nor sleeping properly. He certainly was not exercising regularly, and he was so wrapped up in work that his social life had become virtually nonexistent.

When Rick first experienced respiratory difficulties, his first thought was, quite reasonably, that he had come down with a cold. He didn't pay much attention to it. He just kept on working. When the cold became worse, he decided it had progressed to bronchitis. Convinced that this was the case, he went to see the doctor, took a round of antibiotics, and expected to get well without delay.

Instead of recovering, however, he began to suffer from various allergy symptoms. He continued to work long hours, but he worked with a runny nose and he was constantly sneezing. After coping with two weeks of what he considered to be an allergy attack, he discovered that he was feeling unusually ill. He realized something more was wrong but simply decided his bronchitis had deteriorated into the flu. When what he thought was the flu did not run its normal course, his doctor recommended that he see an allergist.

The allergist did extensive and thorough testing and decided to treat the bronchitis. He also diagnosed candida-related problems and put Rick on a yeast-free diet. He prescribed megavitamins and started a regime of weekly allergy injections. Rick knew he had been allergic to cats when he was a child. He had also suffered from occasional seasonal allergies like ragweed, but he had never suffered from any other serious allergies. He certainly had never dealt with anything that would compare with the difficulties he now faced. "I was still able to go to work," he said. "But it was easy to see that I was getting progressively worse. Although I had always been fortunate enough to have a lot of energy, I developed severe and unexplained exhaustion. I was tired all the time for no particular reason. No matter what I did, no matter how long I slept, I became more and more exhausted until I was so totally drained I would have to go to bed and stay there for days at a time."

Rick's blood tests were positive for Epstein-Barr virus. He was diagnosed with chronic fatigue syndrome. And he again developed bronchial problems that no amount of medication seemed to help.

Discouraged after nine months of continual illness, Rick knew he had to find something that would turn his condition around. He visited a naturopath on the advice of a friend. The naturopath also diagnosed bronchial problems, candida-related problems, and Epstein-Barr virus, which Rick already knew he had. The naturopath added one important item to his diagnosis. He told Rick he was suffering from radiation exposure from his intensive work with computers.

Even though he was constantly exhausted, Rick tried to hold on as best he could to the normal routine of his life. In addition to the long hours he spent working at his full-time job, he owned a business that he was remodeling during nights and weekends. He was putting in new floors, paints, wallpaper, furnishings, and other decorations.

"It was only few weeks after I started seeing the naturopath that I had a very severe reaction to the chemicals in the construction materials," Rick said. "It happened after I had been working with the construction material for three weeks straight. I went to bed one night and could not get up the next morning," he explained. "I couldn't stand. I couldn't walk. I couldn't move. In fact, I was so sick I had to stay in bed for the next two months."

Although he had been seriously ill, Rick's courage and determination to live a normal life had propelled him forward. For months he had been able to function in spite of his sickness, but the exposure to the chemicals in the construction materials was the last straw. His body was no longer able to cope with the load. It was no longer possible for him to maintain even the semblance of a normal life.

"I didn't think that something as normal as a simple remodeling project would be so dangerous to my health. I didn't know what I was doing when I naively exposed myself to the chemicals in the construction materials, but they were just enough to push me over the edge," he explained. Although Rick didn't understand what was happening to him at the time, his immune system had been continually getting worse. He became bedridden. The naturopath ordered homeopathic medicines, which cleared his bronchitis. His allergies were relieved to some degree, but the constant fatigue remained.

"I was determined to improve. I went through every kind of treatment you could possibly think of—colonics, vitamin supplements, diets, homeopathics. Even with all of that, I was only able to go back to work part time. But after I started doing ozone therapy with the naturopathic doctor, I saw enough of an improvement that I was able to be productive at work again. From that point forward I saw cyclical ups and downs. As I gradually improved, I began to see a slow but general trend upward. I dared to begin to think I might improve. I dared to have hope that I was going to get better."

Despite all his attempts, nine months later he suffered a severe relapse. He had moved to another community and no longer had access to the ozone therapy that had helped him so dramatically. He continued to work part time, but he was severely stressed by the knowledge that he wasn't producing the kind or quality of work he wanted to do, the sort of work he had previously been capable of doing. "Remember, I had been a workaholic who had no life outside of work. Perhaps I needed to find balance in my life," he said. "Perhaps I can find some good to have come out of this after all."

Even though Rick wasn't able to accomplish the quality of work he wanted to, at least he was no longer bedridden. He found hope in that. He had no choice but to cut his lifestyle to the bare minimum. "In addition to my full-time job, I had been running my business, and I also had some real estate I was developing. I was forced to cut it all back in order to cope with my illness," he said. "There were times when I would have to go home from work to take a nap, then I would go back to work to finish what I was doing. I was a young guy, but I felt as though I was an old man. That's because I was leading the lifestyle of an old man. During that time I was existing, but I could not say that I was really living."

Rick became severely depressed during the first two years of his illness when he was unable to work, unable to think, unable to do anything but suffer. "Back then, there wasn't even one day when I wanted to be alive," he said. "I got so down during this process I even attempted suicide. After that happened I realized that I had no choice as far as my work was concerned. I needed to take a medical leave of absence from the corporation to address the problem of my declining health."

The corporation refused to grant his leave of absence. "I spoke with all the doctors they wanted me to talk to," he said, the disappointment and disbelief still strongly evident in his voice. "And every one of them told me there was absolutely nothing wrong with me. They told me they had diagnosed nothing. I was barely able to function, and they were telling me there was nothing wrong with me. They were telling me that it was all psychological, that none of the blood work, none of my tests had shown anything wrong. I asked them why, if nothing was wrong with me, I felt so bad. They couldn't answer that. That was not their problem. They had test results on paper, and because of those test results, they wouldn't believe that I was sick. They insisted it was all psychological. I now know that I was dealing with the same old story that so many other people have gone through, but I didn't know it at the time."

What he did know was that he simply could not continue as he was. A competitive man who set high standards for himself, he was no longer productive. When he was able to work, he was not producing the sort of work he was proud of. He decided that he had no choice. If the company would not grant him a leave of absence, there was nothing for him to do but to leave and try to restore his health.

After seeing several more doctors, he found his way to the Great Smokies Medical Center in Asheville, North Carolina. "They did a hair analysis and a mercury-challenged test, and they diagnosed me with mercury toxidity," he said. "I don't know where the mercury came from. It could have come from the food I was eating. It could have come from the water supply. My body had high levels of mercury, aluminum, and lead, but it had toxic levels of mercury."

Rick had all the mercury fillings removed from his teeth. He went through a year's program of getting the mercury taken out of his body. "Having all of your fillings yanked out of your teeth and replaced might sound painful, and it was," he admitted. "But the whole thing is painful. This disease hurts you every way—physically, emotionally, spiritually, and financially."

Rick finally accepted the fact that he wasn't going to be cured in a week or a month or even a year. He admits that he had been fairly headstrong. He had been determined to find a miracle cure, something that would restore his health instantly. He didn't find a miracle. There were no miracles to be found; but he did see gradual improvement. Again he dared to hope. "Although I had reached a level where I wasn't in constant pain, I never had a day where I was completely free of pain, a day when my head was totally clear, or a day when I had any kind of strength. I never felt right. Still, I was able to exist. I could think clearly at times, and I could still enjoy reading at times, although my memory was shot and I couldn't retain anything I read. I found myself at a place of contentment, where I wasn't as sick as I had been but I wasn't anywhere close to as well as I wanted to be."

Although he hated to do it, Rick was forced to apply for Social Security Disability. "I was too sick to work, and I knew I would have to be in treatment for a long time. There's a whole story there, where they always deny you disability until years and years go by. Here again, I now know that many people have gone through the same thing, but I didn't know it then. I lived with my family during that year. As wonderful as they were to me, living with your family is not the ideal situation for a grown man who has been out on his own."

A friend of Rick's who owned a townhouse in Atlanta accepted a job that required constant travel. He suggested that Rick live in his town house and watch it for him when he was away. It worked out to be a win-win situation. His friend had found a reliable housesitter, and Rick had found an acceptable place to live. Rick moved to Atlanta. "That was when I started seeing Dr. Edelson," he said. "The first thing he did was to put me through all the different allergy tests. He discovered that, as a result of the multiple chemical sensitivity, I had become almost universally allergic to foods. I tested allergic to eighty-five out of one hundred foods. I was still sensitive to 40 or 50 percent of the chemicals tested, but not nearly as allergic as I had become to food."

Early in his illness Rick had become aware that it was necessary for him to avoid many of the commonly used household chemicals that provoked reactions. He was careful to stay away not just from household chemicals but from all kinds of chemicals. He believes this may be one reason he didn't develop more extreme chemical sensitivities. However, it's impossible to completely avoid food. A person has to eat. He was eating organic foods, juicing, and was careful to maintain satisfactory nutritional balance. But in spite of all those precautions, his body still developed sensitivities to everything he was eating.

"I went through all the preparation work to do the enzyme potentiated desensitization (EPD) treatments. EPD is a technique where small doses of allergens are used to desensitize you against your own allergies," he explained. "It uses an enzyme called beta glucuronidase, which is found naturally in most humans and animals. What it does is simulate the development of changes in the immune system. When it's used over a long time, sometimes even several years, EPD helps cure allergies to foods, inhalants, and chemicals in about 80 percent of the people who use it. At first you get the vaccine once every two months. After that, the doctor will change the frequency according to your needs. Although there are no serious side effects, you have to follow a really rigid process, and you have to follow instructions carefully and never forget or skip doing those things that are needed to make it work. Before you even start on this program of therapy, the doctor will tell you that you have to be totally committed to getting well and you have to be willing to follow all of the instructions. Well, of course I have always been totally committed to getting well, and I've gotten pretty good at following instructions."

Rick said that within two days after starting the treatments, he felt a remarkable change. "It was the difference between night and day, between light and dark. I felt that dramatic difference for about two weeks. Then after two weeks had passed, I could feel myself slowly start to decline back down to where I had been until it was time for another treatment. After the fourth treatment, I had four weeks where I felt fantastic. I've never achieved that total euphoria again, but as long as I take the EPD treatments, I no longer show the food sensitivities. When I am taking the EPD treatments, I don't suffer from the food allergies or even from the seasonal allergies that caused me so much harm. When it gets to the point where I feel that I am declining, I know I have to go in and have another treatment. I recently tried to push the envelope, to see how far I could go between treatments. That wasn't such a good idea because when I waited too long, I found myself going into a declining process. With the EPD shots, I can almost eat like a normal person. I still have periods of fatigue. I still have the leaky gut, the adrenal problems, and the liver problems, but I have a clear head and my mind is clear now."

Rick has been able to go back to work at least part time for short periods of time. "I have hope that as I improve these short periods of time can get longer. There have been periods when I've been able to go back to work for three months, working half days, sometimes even more and feeling fine. Then I'll have months where I'm struggling to get anything done and to be productive. During those times, I'm not feeling completely terrible, but I can't seem to reach that level of mental sharpness that I need in order to do the intense thinking and concentration I consider necessary for the work I do."

Rick has been sick for a total of nine years. He's realistic about his problems, but he is now hopeful for the future. He has accepted where he is in the evolution of his disease, and he tries to be happy with the considerable progress he has made. "I've come a long way from the time I was confined to bed," he said. "And I'll continue to try to do everything I can to help myself improve. I continue all the diets, the vitamins, the ozone, the EPD, everything that's necessary. At this point, I feel that I'm in control of my illness. Even though I'm not strong, and I don't have any times of peak energy, I don't suffer from the truly bad times either. I don't suffer from the mood swings or the depression."

Rick has come into contact with people who were far worse than he is. He described some truly tragic stories, saying that nothing seems to help some people. He has averaged ten to fifteen thousand dollars a year in medical-related costs, none of it covered by insurance, but he considers himself lucky to have had sufficient financial resources to try everything and anything that might help him improve. "I was fortunate to have a loving family that wouldn't give up on me," he said. "No matter how bad I was, no matter how discouraged I was or how discouraged they were, even when I was suicidal, they never turned away from me. I was fortunate to have caring friends who were willing to help me. And I know there's a lot of prayer that's helped me too. Certainly, my spiritual faith has helped me to climb up out of my depression, to come back from the darkness of a time when I no longer wanted to live."

Despite all he's been through, Rick looks for the positive side of his illness. "Before I got sick I was a committed workaholic. I have always been a spiritual person, but I'd even quit going to church because I was so busy at work. I didn't socialize because I was so wrapped up in my work. I didn't date because I was so wrapped up in my work. I needed a change of direction. I needed to learn how to appreciate even the smallest things life has to offer. Now, I'm thankful for every meal I eat when I'm able to eat it. I appreciate this country and the freedoms we have. I appreciate our many blessings."

One of the positives Rick mentions with pride is the fact that he met his wife Kaye at Dr. Edelson's office. "Dr. Edelson is an unlikely cupid, and his office is an unlikely place to meet your true love," Rick said. "But love is where you find it."

Kaye also suffers from multiple chemical sensitivity. "We were both in chelation therapy. When you're hooked up to an IV for two or three hours, you talk to anyone who'll listen to you. Kaye was really having a bad day. I understood her problems. I also know from my own experience that sometimes the smallest ray of hope can help a person make it through the day, or even through the hour. It bothered her that she wasn't able to work. When she said she worked with computers, I told her we could find a way to overcome that. That evening I went out to her house and set up her home computer to see if she might be able to do some work from home. We had a nice visit, and we discovered we had a lot in common besides our chemical sensitivity and our interest in computers. One thing led to another, and things progressed from there. Love can find many doors. Of course, Dr. Edelson was a guest at our wedding."

14

Enzyme Potentiated Desensitization

ENZYME POTENTIATED DESENSITIZATION (EPD) immunotherapy treatment, which helped Rick and others achieve such dramatic improvement, was developed by Dr. Len McEwen, M.D. of
London, England, in the 1960s and has successfully been used in
England since that time.

Studies suggest that EPD has much greater long-term success than
any other method of immunotherapy. Useful in the treatment of a
large variety of conditions that were previously considered to be unre-
sponsive to immunotherapy, it has been found to stimulate the development of immune system changes that can, over a period of time,
cure allergies to foods, inhalants, and chemicals in over 80 percent of
the suitable patients.

With EPD, extremely small doses of allergens are used to attempt to
desensitize you to your allergies. Very-low-dose allergens are mixed
with the enzyme beta glucuronidase, which is a natural protein found
in all parts of the human body and throughout the animal kingdom.

Although beta glucuronidase is an enzyme, it appears to have a second function that allows it to serve as a messenger in the immune system. It has the ability to stimulate the body to become tolerant to an allergen that is administered at the same time in an extremely small, safe dose. Although the quantity of the enzyme necessary for the treatment could be extracted from a few cc's of human blood, the highly purified substance that is used is actually extracted from the digestive gland of the abalone, a large sea mollusk.

In situations of ordinary environmental exposure, when an allergen enters your body and provokes symptoms, the dose of allergen will be enough to excite increased sensitivity as well. This effect is augmented by the large quantity of beta glucuronidase liberated by the allergic response. EPD decreases this sensitivity by delivering accurate, ultra-low doses of allergens—far less than would enter the body from ordinary environmental exposure—combined with a small, precise dose of beta glucuronidase.

Instead of "shouting" and provoking symptoms, the small, controlled EPD "whispers" a natural message to the immune system and generates a new family of cells. After three weeks, when they are mature, these cells travel throughout the body actively switching off allergies. The immune system that had failed and allowed the allergy to develop is gradually restored to normal self-regulation.

Since EPD uses one of nature's own pathways to activate a natural regulatory process, its effects are easily influenced by the body's hormones, nutrition, and environment. Drugs are not susceptible to these factors in the same way and neither are the effects of treatments.

The advantages of EPD over other treatments are numerous. It is the only potentially curative immunotherapy for allergies. It can be cost effective over a period of years. It is more convenient than conventional immunotherapies which demand more frequent injections. The vaccine is made in the doctor's office using readily available components. Also, it involves only minimal, temporary dietary restrictions, and after those discomforts, it offers the hope of eating normally again in the future. Since the dose of allergen needed is much smaller than that used for conventional desensitization injections, this treatment is also considerably safer.

Two methods of EPD are in current use. The cup method is sometimes used for children and other people who do not like to take injections. The cup method involves scarification of a small area of the forearm or thigh to remove the waterproof layer of the skin. A plastic cup is then taped in place to hold the desensitizing fluid over the scarification for twenty-four hours. The slow absorption of the dose makes this exceptionally safe. In addition, the immune system is much more reactive to agents that reach it through the skin than it is to ordinary injections.

The second method is by intradermal injection. A fine needle is introduced into the skin of the forearm. The injection is absorbed into the system slowly through the same channels that would be reached by the cup method. EPD has been successfully used in treating asthma, rhinitis, nasal polyps, eczema, urticaria, irritable bowel syndrome, migraines, rheumatoid arthritis, petit mal epilepsy, psychiatric reactions to food, and chemical sensitivity, including reactions to fumes and smells. Also, the secondary allergies that complicate post-viral syndrome (CFS) often respond to EPD.

Although most recognized allergies are suitable for treatment, unfortunately, not every allergy is suitable. At present, EPD has not been developed for treatment of contact dermatitis, aspirin allergy, allergy to other drugs, or allergy to stinging insects. It is limited in its effectiveness against chemical additives in foods because of the great number and variety of chemicals used by the food industry, but most of the important food colors and preservatives are included. EPD may be helpful if food intolerance is involved in other illnesses, even when the cause of the condition remains difficult to determine. Even though the treatment of allergy to outdoor molds is likely to be successful, allergy to mold spores inside a damp house is often impossible to treat because of the vast number of mold species that can thrive in such circumstances.

Desensitizing mixtures are available to treat sensitivities to a wide variety of inhalants such as pollens, dust, pet hair and dander, natural foods, food additives, candida, and fumes from perfumes and cosmetics. When EPD is used, many allergens cross-desensitize in groups. To allow for this, representative allergens have been chosen to ensure the widest possible effect.

Allergen mixtures are used in EPD for several reasons. Many patients are sensitive to a wider range of allergens than they may consciously recognize. Allergy sufferers who are not treated by EPD tend to recruit new sensitivities with time. There is solid evidence that EPD with mixed allergens protects against this problem. Also, allergens absorbed from the environment near the time of EPD are part of the treatment. It is better to take control by including effective doses in the injection.

How frequently EPD treatment is necessary depends on a person's individual need and the type and severity of his allergy. Frequency will be decided after a thorough consultation, including a complete history, physical examination, and laboratory evaluation. Before starting on a course of EPD, it is important to be certain of the diagnosis, the nutritional health of the patient, and any other complicating factors. EPD will not work in a person who is not nutritionally sound.

Initial doses tend to be given at two- to three-month intervals for the first year or two of treatment. After the response is well established, the frequency of the desensitization can be diminished to between one and three each year. Some people have received doses over a period of up to twenty years without ill effects. More than half the people treated with EPD have been able to stop treatment for long intervals without suffering ill effects. The longest recorded interval was twenty-one years.

Although the full benefit of EPD may be slow to appear, the effect of EPD treatment can be almost immediate. The response to EPD has four distinct phases:

1. *Reaction Time.* Up to three weeks, during which time an immediate "cure" for symptoms may result.

2. *Main Action.* This begins after three to four weeks and usually lasts three to four months. Later doses may last up to one year.

3. *Late Response.* This can occur from one-and-a-half to two-and-a-half years and seven to nine doses after the start of treatment.

4. *Postponed Action.* This appears between six and fifteen months after the final dose of an adequate course of EPD. It is often a permanent cure.

If nine doses of EPD have been given over two-and-a-half years with no obvious benefit, the doctor will stop treatment in order to allow this last action sufficient time to develop.

As Rick explained in the previous chapter, the preparation for EPD treatment is very specific. Before you start on this particular program of therapy, your doctor will explain that you have to be totally committed to getting well and that you have to be willing to follow all of the instructions rigidly and without any changes or exceptions. It is important that you be completely committed to the program because the regimen you will be required to follow involves a truly rigid process. It will be necessary for you to follow instructions carefully and never forget to do those things that are needed to make the desensitization work.

Just like the long, involved questionnaire and the seemingly nosey conversation you had when you first visited your environmental physician, there is, of course, a reason for everything you will be asked to do during the course of EPD treatment. The involved question- naire helped your doctor find out about you while, at the same time, it helped you focus on the problem areas in your life. The long, nosey conversation with your doctor helped her learn more about you and helped you discover seemingly unrelated events and activities that turned out to have a direct bearing on your health problems. In the same way, strict adherence to the EPD regimen is not only reasonable, it is vital to the success of your treatment.

If you accidentally take in too much allergen from other sources, the "whispered" message of EPD can be transformed into a "shout" and it can reverse the effect for the allergen that is concerned. The highest risk of this happening occurs during the first twenty-four hours after you have had the EPD treatment. After a week has passed, it will be harder to upset the treatment in this particular way.

However, when the message of the treatment has successfully been delivered, the developing family of suppresser cells can be diverted by several kinds of natural or manmade stimuli. Since it will take three weeks for them to mature, it will be necessary for you to continue to observe certain rules and guidelines during this significant length of time. There are rules of restricted activity, restricted diet, water con- sumption, medications, and even your surroundings. At first these rules may seem to be confusing or even frightening, but after careful consideration you will realize that they are simply based on common sense. Failures of EPD, or reports of symptoms becoming worse or new allergies appearing, have been traced to people who have blatantly ignored the simple restrictions in diet, personal activities, and surroundings.

For at least twenty-four hours before EPD and for two days after the treatment, you will be asked to avoid those allergens that you know can upset you. To avoid provoking hidden inhalant allergies, you will also be asked to avoid large doses of other potential allergens. To do this, you must avoid significant exposure to pollens, molds, pets, and dust, at least for the critical sixty hours after your treatment. During those significant sixty hours you will be asked to keep to the minimum exposure to chemicals and fumes of all kinds, including wood fires and tobacco smoke. To be on the safe side, it would be best for you to also avoid contact with newsprint. And you will certainly want to avoid all those glossy magazines that contain scented advertisements.

You should drink plenty of water every day during the first week. A minimum of a pint of water four times a day is recommended, and more water is recommended during hot weather.

There is a good reason for doing this. The hormone vasopressin, which reduces urine volume when you are thirsty, also acts as a messenger in the immune system and can reverse the effect of treatment during the first six days after EPD. This can be avoided by drinking plenty of water.

If your doctor advises you to do so, you should take standard vitamin therapy including zinc, folic acid, vitamins A and D, multivitamins, and minerals. If you are instructed to do so, by all means you should take your course of antifungal or antibacterial drugs before EPD. If you are trying to become pregnant, it would be best to have EPD during the first two weeks after a period and avoid vitamin A and misoprostol (Cytotec).

It is best not to have a dose of EPD during the first five days of a cold, or if you have any other infection or suspect you might be developing an infection. However, if you have had a bacterial infection such as bronchitis, you should discuss your situation with your doctor. Bronchitis that has been treated with antibiotics and is well on the way to a cure may be acceptable.

You certainly don't want to have a dose of EPD if you think you may be pregnant. Don't have a dose of EPD if you have just been immunized, if you have an appointment for dental treatment scheduled during the two-and-a-half weeks after the EPD treatment, if you are wearing scent, if you have recently put ointment of any kind on or near the place where the dose of EPD will be administered, or if you have taken any pain killer (such as aspirin or acetaminophen) during the three days before the treatment. If you know that you are food sensitive, you must diet as instructed by your doctor before taking the dose. If you or your doctor believe you might be food sensitive, or if you have ever suffered from problems such as eczema, urticaria, or angio-edema, psychological depression, migraines, epilepsy, irritable bowel, Crohn's disease, ulcerative colitis, arthritis, or lupus, it would be best to follow the basic EPD diet for at least twelve hours before EPD and twenty-four hours afterward to avoid possible food allergies. Do not have a dose of EPD if you have not dieted as instructed. If you are allergic to candida, you will be required to do a preliminary "gut preparation." Do not take the dose of EPD if you have neglected to do this.

There are certain factors and seemingly simple events that can upset the effectiveness of EPD treatment. Although you are usually safe after two weeks, influenza or other troublesome infections can be harmful if you come down with them soon after your EPD treatment. If possible, it is best to avoid physical or mental stress at the time of treatment and at least one week afterward. Physical stress appears to be less harmful than a severe mental shock. Excessive sexual activity is best avoided for a few days. Dental treatment is best avoided within one week before or two-and-a-half weeks after treatment.

Various contraceptive pills and other female hormone preparations, particularly implants, can also affect EPD.

Vitamin C in very high doses (30 gm or more taken intravenously) may wipe out the effect of EPD at any time. More than 500 mg a day may reduce the overall success during the three weeks after EPD. As little as one gm a day has caused EPD to fail. Although it seems to be contradictory, if you take two to three gm of vitamin C a day for two weeks and stop twenty-four hours prior to EPD, you may improve the response.

If you are not acclimated to conditions of extreme heat, you will find this can adversely affect EPD. Many kinds of toiletries, skin treatments, domestic chemicals, and chemicals at work can also have an adverse effect on EPD, as can the type of copper bracelet that is sometimes worn as a remedy for arthritis.

It is important to know that heavy exposure to any aerosol such as perfume, polish, paint spray, or hair spray in a confined space within twenty-four hours of EPD can provoke an attack of asthma, whether or not you have ever suffered from asthma before. Fortunately, such accidents have not resulted in permanent asthma.

Watch Your Medications and Drugs

Certain drugs can upset the success of EPD, although there are often temporary ways to avoid problems with medications. Be sure that your environmental physician understands every medication you are putting on or into your body before you begin your EPD treatment. Please remember that herbal medicines can be powerful drugs and may also influence the results of EPD. Evening primrose oil, other gamma linolenic acid (GLA) preparations, and flax seed should not be taken near the time of treatment. Also, some vitamins and other supplements such as royal jelly can effect EPD.

Even a single dose of Nalcrom (disodium cromoglycate, cromolyn sodium) taken by mouth appears to destroy the effect of EPD. Never use Nalcrom before four weeks after EPD treatment. Even at that time never use the drug more often than once each week. Digestive enzymes can sometimes offer partial protection from food allergies if they are taken immediately before a meal and should be used in place of Nalcrom.

For four days before EPD and three weeks afterward, you must avoid the antibacterial sulfonamides, trimethoprim, or combinations of the two. Septra is the most common, although their are many trade names. You must also avoid large doses of anti-asthmatic drugs, particularly by inhalation, Ventolin, or related drugs for asthma by mouth, injection, or nebulizer. In some instances, aerosols or inhaled powders may be acceptable.

Avoid most over-the-counter pain killing drugs, particularly aspirin, Tylenol, Motrin, and other nonsteroidal, anti-inflammatory drugs. This is a group comprised mostly of drugs used to relieve mild to moderate pain, fever, menstrual pains, and as first-line treatment for arthritis. Nearly forty brands can be prescribed and many more can be bought over the counter without a prescription. NSAIDs must be avoided for three and a half weeks after EPD because even a single dose taken during that time is likely to reverse the treatment. Your doctor will know special ways of dealing with your particular problem if it is essential that you take an NSAID for arthritis, or aspirin to protect against blood clots.

Avoid diet pills of any kind as well as all cold cures and nasal decongestants whether they are taken by mouth or used in the nose, and avoid antimalarial drugs. Substitute omeprazole (Losec) for Zantac, Tagamet, or similar stomach ulcer drugs.

Large doses of estrogens, such as implants used for contraception, birth control pills, and post-menopausal hormone therapy, are likely to interfere with EPD. Small doses in the "mini" contraceptive pills and low-dose HRT will not interfere.

Large doses of progesterone are druglike and may suppress allergy symptoms. Progesterone itself does not usually worsen allergies but should not be given at the same time as EPD. This is particularly true of implants. Synthetic progesterone derivatives are used in contraceptive pills to provoke "false periods" for protection against cancer, and they are used in high doses to treat menstrual irregularities and premenstrual tension. Most of them will make allergies worse and interfere with EPD.

Danol (Danazol) is a sex-hormonelike drug used to suppress the female hormone cycle. It is exceptionally likely to worsen allergies and is incompatible with EPD.

In addition to these prescription and over-the-counter drugs, all illegal drugs, including marijuana, can cause your allergy to return at any time.

There are certain drugs that do not seem to upset EPD. They include cortisone and its related medications; antidepressants, except MAOIs and tranquilizers; antihistamines of the kind used for hay fever; blood pressure drugs; diuretics; antibiotics other than those mentioned above; prescription pain killers; Theyphylline and its relatives used for asthma; disodium cromoglycate (Intal) used for asthma except when taken by mouth as Nalcrom; and ergotamine/caffeine used for migraine.

Temporary Changes in Your Personal Hygiene Habits

Your physician will give you a list of personal rules and regulations for temporary changes in your personal hygiene habits. You are to observe these rules conscientiously.

Ointments, creams, and lotions are to be avoided on any part of the body during the day before and the day after EPD. They should not be used on the arm that has been treated with EPD for a full week after the treatment. In fact, you will be asked not even to use the hand of the arm that has been treated with EPD to apply these preparations to other parts of the body. If it is necessary to do so you will be asked to cover the hand with a protective glove.

Your bathing, washing, and toiletry habits may be temporarily amended. You will be asked to use only simple soap or its equivalent the day before and the full week after EPD. Avoid using bath oil, liquid soap, body bath, or powder, particularly on the hand of the treated arm. Do not use hair sprays, conditioners, or hair oils, mousse, gel, or spritzes. Use no shampoo until at least four days after EPD, then only use "simple shampoo" for two weeks. Do not use toothpaste the day before or the day after EPD. Use no deodorant, not even unscented deodorant for three days before and one week after EPD. Substitute unscented talcum. Use no permanent waving, hair color, or other extensive hair treatments the week before and the three weeks after EPD and stay out of the beauty shop completely. Men will not use shaving gel, shaving cream, or aftershave lotion. Instead, they may use an electric razor. Women will keep make-up to a minimum and be sure they do not use perfumed make-up.

Temporary Changes in Your Activities

Your normal routine of athletic activity is not likely to interfere with EPD after the first few days, but you should avoid exercising to the point of physical fatigue for at least ten days. Obviously, this is not the time to decide to run the marathon, to dance *Swan Lake*, or to enter an aerobics competition. If you suffer from complex illnesses, you should avoid exercising to the point of physical fatigue until two weeks after EPD. People who suffer from post-viral fatigue syndrome should never exercise to the point of fatigue.

Avoid becoming overheated for a week after your EPD treatment. However, if you live in a hot climate and are already accustomed to very hot weather, the heat will not affect your treatment. During the week after EPD, do not take hot baths and do not use a sauna. Although sunbathing more than five days before EPD is likely to offer you some advantage, you should avoid becoming particularly hot while sunbathing during the week after EPD, and do not do anything that will heat the arm that received the treatment.

Control Your Surroundings

Of course, we all understand it would be impossible for you to completely control everything in your surroundings at home, at work, and while you are traveling, but you will want to do the best you can to stay away from offending allergens.

At work

If you have been upset by allergens at work, it would be best to take the EPD treatments when you can be away from work and remain away from work for several days. You will probably want to arrange for EPD treatment near the weekend or at a time when you can comfortably use at least twenty-four hours to as much as three days of your sick time or vacation time. When you return to work, avoid inhaling tobacco smoke from other people's cigars, cigarettes, and pipes. Avoid other people's perfume and perfumed products. Avoid air-conditioned offices with recirculated air, particularly if you suspect "sick building" or "tight building" problems. Avoid humidified work places, particularly printing plants. Stay away from modern industrial processes that generate fumes, such as plastics, fiberglass, soldering, paint shops, chemical processing plants, and foundries. If your work is in agriculture, stay away from dusty work, damp environments, feedstuffs, livestock, and chemicals. Avoid coming into contact with newsprint, paper that has a shiny finish or any recognizable odor, old books, and dusty or damp paper such as those found in some offices and basements. Stay away from most office machinery, including photocopiers, fax machines, computers, and printers.

At home

It is important for you to stay away from mold spores. Sometimes the mold that is in flowerpots or on indoor plants may cause allergies, and sometimes the house plants themselves are allergens. Spores from ferns and scents emanating from leaves or flowers can cause problems. It may be best to put your houseplants outdoors or send your houseplants "on vacation" to a friend's or relative's home while you are preparing for and undergoing EPD, and by all means tell those who care for you that this is not a good time to send you flowers. Remove all potpourri from your surroundings because it is scented and it always contains mold spores.

Houses that are continually damp; suffer from condensation; smell musty or even have a small area that was once damp in particular rooms or cupboards; and cellars and basements will have high concentrations of mold spores floating in the air. These mold spores stay in the air indefinitely. Some other significant sources of mold spores can include old stored vegetables as well as outdoor clothing that has not dried properly.

If your house has a damp room or cellar, simply keeping the door shut will not afford you effective protection from mold spores, which float easily through the air. Your exposure may be reduced by good, thorough ventilation both night and day. Use an ozone unit to clean the rooms. If this is not possible or if it is not practical and if you know that your house contains damp areas, you must leave before, during and shortly after EPD. Stay with someone who has a dry, modern, dust-free house with no pets the day before and two days after EPD.

You will choose to severely restrict yourself from contact with domestic chemicals at least twelve hours before and two to four days after EPD. Avoid newsprint and printer's ink. Stay away from aerosols, spray polishes, and perfumed sprays, scents, and air fresheners of any kind. Avoid the smell of new paint. Avoid smelling scented or biological washing powders and lavatory cleaners of all kinds. Keep away from scented sheets, towels, and bathroom supplies. Avoid new carpets, new vinyl wallpaper, new furniture, and new plastic sheeting such as shower curtains, table covers, and furniture covers.

Remember, some domestic items such as vinyl wallpaper give off fumes that can cause problems even though they are virtually odorless. As they get older, they will give off fewer fumes and become safer.

You will want to keep out of stores that sell perfumes, washing powders, fabrics, furnishings, carpets, newspapers, and books for some length of time after EPD.

Do not breathe any insecticides that produce vapor or might be inhaled, such as sprays, aerosols, smokes, blocks, mothballs, and clothing preservatives. Do not use hanging pest strips. You may use ordinary flypaper, which is resin coated but contains no insecticide. If it is absolutely necessary to control roaches during this time, use one of the proprietary flea powders that are produced for use on cats and dogs. These do not vaporize. Ask another person to puff it into cracks where the insects hide. This protection is long lasting and is not likely to harm you. Boric acid products are also useful and effective.

Travel

It is possible to be successfully and safely treated with EPD even though you are obliged to ride in cars, buses, trains, and airplanes in order to reach your doctor's office for your treatment. With the exception of rare occasions, the doses of allergens you might inhale during your trip is generally too small to upset the treatment. Some obvious and simple precautions can help protect you.

Try not to inhale excessive doses of "fumes" from other people's scents, newspapers, magazines, papers, and ink as well as from the traffic itself. If you are driving during the spring and summer months, keep your car windows shut to avoid breathing high doses of pollens from the roadside. Normal, limited exposure to exhaust fumes is not likely to harm you even if it provokes symptoms, but avoid riding with a leaking exhaust. Avoid riding in new cars with smelly interiors. Also, avoid riding in old cars with moldy carpets and seats. If you are riding on public transportation, don't sit next to a smoker or a to heavily perfumed passenger.

Diet and EPD

If you are food sensitive, you must diet carefully at the time of EPD. The EPD diet is extremely limited and extremely restricted, but you can take comfort from knowing that you will not have to remain on it very long. The critical time for the extremely restricted EPD treatment diet is the twenty-four hours before EPD and up to forty-eight hours afterward. Since an excessive intake of a food allergen that is important to you may upset the treatment, it will probably be wise for you to follow a post-EPD diet as well. Many food allergens cross-react in the desensitizing process, so it is not safe to only avoid those foods that give you symptoms or those to which you are positive in any kind of test.

Basic EPD treatment diet

Although this diet seems harsh, it is very simple. It contains only foods that are likely to be safe. No matter how sorely you may be tempted to do so, do not add snacks, sweets, sauces, flavorings, or drinks not listed on the diet. Do not add anything to it. Do not change it in any way except after discussion with your doctor. You should eat only these things:

Meat: Lamb, rabbit, some white fish, venison

Starch: Potatoes, sweet potatoes, yams, tapioca (cassava), sago

Vegetables: Cooked carrots, parsnips, rutabagas, celery, cabbage, lettuce. Use only the outside leaves of celery, cabbage, and lettuce, not the hearts.

Fruit: Rhubarb (fresh or frozen). Do not use rhubarb that has been colored. You can use a little bicarbonate of soda to reduce the acidity of cooked rhubarb. If you use too much, your food will taste salty. For a sweet taste, add a little fructose.

Fat for cooking: You may use lamb fat and drippings and small quantities of sunflower oil.

Drinks: Bottled spring water, either flat or sparkling. (Be sure to drink at least eight glasses of water every day.)

Other: Fructose for sweetening, pure baking soda, sea salt that does not include an additive so that it can be "free running."

It is important to remember that herbs and spices cross-react with other foods. They must be avoided while you are on this diet. If you believe you might be sensitive to any of these foods, they must be kept out of your diet.

Fructose-only diet

People who have multiple and complex food allergies often respond to EPD best if they take in only fructose and spring water for forty-eight hours at the time of treatment. The fructose will stave off hunger and protect against hypoglycemia, but it is not intended to replace the calories in a normal diet. A dose of one to two teaspoons of fructose every hour or two is sufficient. The quantity is not critical, but too much fructose will give you diarrhea.

You may take the fructose plain by the spoonful of dry powder or you may stir it into spring water. It is extremely sweet. This extreme sweetness can prove to be unpleasant to some people. A better way to take it is to freeze a strong solution of fructose in spring water to make a kind of sorbet, which can be eaten by the spoonful and washed down with water.

Fructose is a sugar used by diabetics. Unlike other sugars, fructose offers a slow, steady supply of energy and protects against hypoglycemia (low blood sugar.) Fructose can feed the bacteria and yeasts that cause the jejunal fermentation syndrome, but everyone who suffers with this must be treated with a "gut preparation," usually of antifungal drug and bismuth, to clear out these organisms before each treatment of EPD.

Although fructose may be manufactured from corn starch, the dose of corn allergen it contains is too small to provoke significant symptoms, so that it does not interfere with desensitization to corn. It can be purchased in health food stores.

The eat-nothing diet

Before the fructose-only diet was introduced, people were expected to fast completely, eating nothing and drinking only spring water. This was continued for two full days at the time of EPD. Although this was successful for many people, the result of each shot of EPD can be less reliable since the stress of an attack of hypoglycemia can upset the treatment.

The four-day post-EPD diet

During the week that follows the strict EPD diet, a tiny quantity of food to which you are allergic will not harm you, although a large quantity prevents desensitization to that food as well as to other foods related to it. There are three ways to manage your diet successfully. If you are only sensitive to a limited number of foods, just avoid those foods that cause you to have problems.

Remain on the limited EPD diet which you were on during the time of treatment, and add small portions of additional foods to widen your diet. Be careful to avoid foods that previously upset you.

If you react to many foods and were severely restricted or used only fructose at treatment time, you will not be obliged to eat foods that your immune system can recognize as allergens. The intake of each food must be extremely small in order to avoid upsetting the effect of EPD. This means you will be eating doses, rather than portions of each food. To have enough food, you will have to eat tiny quantities of a great many foods at the same time. "The Very Mixed Diet" is the way to do this. You will need to understand it and be prepared for it before you have your dose of EPD.

The very mixed diet

For all immune and allergic reactions, even in a test tube, there is a particular dose of the harmful agent, the antigen or allergen, which causes the maximum reaction. That is the only dose that will do so. A larger dose does nothing. With food reactions, the amount of harmful food eaten is likely to be the amount that causes the maximum trouble. A larger quantity of that same food may cause no reaction at all, particularly if it is eaten once every five days. This is called masking. Masking works independently for each allergen, so that allergies to other foods may still be identified.

Masking can be a satisfactory way to achieve short-term well-being. It is not quite as acceptable as a method of maintaining health for a period of many years, although there is no doubt that it can work effectively for some people.

EPD does not abolish allergies. Instead, it increases the dose of allergen needed to provoke illness by a factor of between tens and thousands. As a result, ordinary exposures to the allergen become harmless. Instead of masking, extra large doses of allergen now begin to cause reactions. As a result of this, you will begin to develop symptoms as the desensitization process progresses if you have been eating a food in a masking dose. The most likely time that you will develop these symptoms is a few weeks after the second or third dose of EPD when the desensitization begins to work.

If this should happen to you, it will be necessary to change your diet and change your whole way of thinking about your food. The question you must face is no longer, "What am I allergic to?" The question you must ask yourself has changed to, "How much of each kind of food can I eat without developing uncomfortable symptoms?"

When this happens, you can get well by eating a tiny quantity of each food, even foods that made you sick in the past. In order to keep down the tiny quantity of each food, you will need to eat many different kinds of food at each meal and you will do this without any rotation. Although this may sound wonderful to you after a long process of carefully controlled rotation dieting, it will not be nearly as easy as it sounds because it is going to require a considerable amount of planning and preparation.

Even so, the new diet will only be a temporary nuisance. Once you are established on the system and you see that your symptoms are improving, you can and should start exploring different foods to discover what you can eat in ordinary quantities. You will no longer be forced to worry about avoiding allergens. Your new concern is how much of a food is it safe for you to eat.

To complicate digestive matters even further, your desensitization is not likely to be stable in the early stages. The safe amounts of your food allergies will increase for a few weeks after treatment, but they will begin to decrease again before you take the next dose. Do not allow this to discourage you. With time, the safe quantities should increase progressively and the result should become stable.

Each section of the Very Mixed Diet is prepared from a carefully chosen mixture of ingredients. You will rely on a grain mixture, like boiled rice or pasta, as a source of energy. You will add meat stew to the grain mixture for a main dish with vegetables. There is a potato mixture that can also be used with the meat. Adding fish to the grain mixture will give you kedgeree, which you may choose to eat for a first course or as a main dish. The same grain mixture can be warmed with milk and sweetening to make a dessert pudding or fruit puree.

Although many of these recipes seem troublesome to prepare, you will find that several days' supply of each mixture may be cooked in advance and frozen in serving portions.

Grain	Proportions by weight
Barley	1
Rye	1
Rice	1
Millet	1
Buckwheat	2
Pearl sago	2

If lentils or soya seeds do not cause you to have problems, you may add one part of lentils or whole soya seeds to the grain mixture for variety in taste and texture. It is best to precook each ingredient separately because the different grains may not cook thoroughly at the same rate. Add a pinch of salt to the cooking water. Strain and mix the grains as they cool.

To prepare a flour that may be baked into biscuits and bread, made into crispbread on an iron bakestone, or fried into thin wafers like Indian chapatis, you will need to add more protein to the grain mixture. For more interesting results in taste and texture you can use the following mixture:

Ingredients	Proportions by weight
Barley flour	1
Rye flour	1
Rice flour	1
Millet flour	1
Soy flour or chickpea flour	1
Buckwheat grits	2
Pearl sago (ground coarsely)	2

The buckwheat grits and particles of sago will give "bite" to preparations made with this flour. You can grind the pearl sago yourself by using a coffee grinder designed for home use. If you cannot obtain buckwheat grits, you may buy whole buckwheat and use the coffee grinder to grind them. If you do not like the rough texture produced by this addition, you may buy buckwheat and sago flours instead.

You may also use this flour to bake bread. The dose of yeast you will receive if you use it to bake bread is so small you should be able to tolerate it without discomfort. If using the yeast should upset you, you may substitute by using baking powder to bake soda bread.

MEAT
Use equal parts of at least four of the following meats:
Beef
Lamb
Pork
Chicken
Venison
Rabbit

You may use the kidney or heart portions of these meats to provide a variety of taste to your meals but you may not use liver.

Cut the meat into small pieces, and grind it or mince it. Fry it in a small amount of corn oil. Add salt to taste. Cook in a small volume of water. The best results will be obtained by cooking it in a covered casserole in the oven.

The flavor may also be improved by adding 1/4 teaspoon of chopped chives for each helping before cooking.

FISH
Use equal portions of each of the following fish:
Cod
Sole
Salmon

Precook the cod and sole. Remove the bones and break into pieces. Although fresh salmon may have a better taste, canned salmon should be satisfactory. If you use canned salmon, drain the water, break the fish into pieces, and mix with the other fish you have cooked in the combination. Freeze small portions for later use.

To make kedgeree, add a serving portion of the fish mixture to a serving of the grain mixture. Stir together and heat thoroughly. Top with margarine. You may use a little parsley.

Potato

Tapioca is really a root vegetable used as an important source of starch, especially in tropical Africa. Its native name is cassava. It is logical to mix it with potato. Use equal parts of these:

> White potato
> Sweet potato
> Tapioca

Cook each ingredient separately. Add a pinch of salt, mash, mix, and freeze portions.

Pea-Carrot Mixture

Use equal parts by volume of the following:

> Peas
> Chopped green beans
> Celery

Add two bunches of carrots

(Many people will not be upset by adding corn on the cob.)

It is best to use fresh vegetables. If it is not possible for you to use fresh vegetables, you can buy frozen packets of each of these ingredients. Mix the different vegetables and return them to the freezer. Avoid brands that contain a lot of artificial color. Remember, carrots and celery are powerful allergens until they are cooked. Once cooked, they are safe for most people.

Tomato Puree

Make your own tomato puree. Cook well. Add salt. If you wish, you may add a small amount of lemon juice or cider vinegar to taste. If it does not upset you, a dash of pepper, mint, or basil may be included. For a different taste, add a small amount of chopped bell pepper before cooking. Freeze small portions.

Since tomato is a strong allergen, it would be best to start by using only a teaspoonful per helping to add flavor to your meals. Do not use tomato or vinegar in any other way during the time you are on this diet.

Fruit Parts by volume

Stew together these items:

Apple	1
Dried banana slices	2
Blackberry or black currant	1
Apricot	1/2
Rhubarb	3

After cooking the fresh vegetables, you may add an extra part of chopped canned peaches, preferably water pack instead of syrup. Add a small amount bicarbonate of soda to neutralize some of the acid. Do not use too much or it will have a salty taste. If necessary, you may sweeten the mixture sparingly with fructose.

Many people will find that a faint flavor of ginger or cinnamon adds variety and interest to the fruit and does not upset them. You may try to add these if you like; it is best to use a pinch of true powdered spice during cooking. Do not use liquid essence from a bottle.

Some meal plans and recipes

If you are preparing a main dish, prepare the grain mixture as a base. Spread the meat mixture over the grain mixture. For variety, you can add a teaspoonful of tomato puree to the meat mixture. Heat and serve.

If you would like to prepare an alternative main dish meal, you can serve the meat mixture with the potato mixture. Form the potato mixture into a round ball and serve the meat mixture on the side. You can add variety to this dish by warming the meat with the pea-carrot mixture instead serving it separately.

Fish can be used in many ways. You may use the fish as a main course and serve it with the vegetable mixture or with the grain or potato mixture. Use the fish kedgeree as an extra course to start the meal. You may be able to tolerate a dash of lemon to season the fish. Fruit puree may be eaten with a small amount of the grain by adding a small amount of Carnation milk. Add just enough Carnation milk to the grain to moisten it and to give it a somewhat creamy texture. The fruit puree may be eaten alone or with a cake made from the mixed flour. Later you may choose to use the Carnation cream recipe as a topping.

Hot cakes can be made by using the flour mixture. Prepare the various flours in the directed proportions. Mix them by weight or by volume.

HOT CAKES
   1 1/3 cups mixed flour
   3 teaspoons baking powder
   pinch of salt
   enough sparkling spring water to moisten the dough (do not make it too runny)

Heat a skillet and grease the surface with a small amount of hard margarine. Drop a tablespoonful of dough on the hot skillet. Fry until brown. This recipe will produce small cakes that can be stored in a tin. They may be frozen for longer storage.

You can create a pastry by using the full grain mixture. You may vary the pastry by eliminating the sago from the flour mixture. Use eight ounces of the flour mixture. Add eight ounces of pure sago flour so that half the total mixture is sago.

PASTRY

> Mix 8 oz. of the sago-mixed grain flour
> 4 oz. hard margarine, softened to room temperature
> pinch of salt
> approximately 2 tablespoons ice water

Preheat oven to 400 degrees F. Sift the flour and salt into a mixing bowl. Cut in the margarine until the mixture looks like fine bread crumbs. Slowly add ice water until mixture clings together. Roll out on a floured board. Cut and use as desired. Bake in the preheated oven for ten to fifteen minutes.

Drinks

Water is the best thing you can drink. Eight glasses of water every day is essential. Various kinds of spring waters are good for you.

Plain tea in tea bags is acceptable. You may experiment with tea mixtures, but remember that the true teas contain a stimulant drug. A mixture of herbal tea and ordinary China tea can offer a pleasant alternative to your limited choice of beverages. Add 2/3 part chamomile tea and 1/3 part China blend tea. A mixture of equal parts of Keemun and Lapsang Souchong makes a nice China tea.

Coffee should be avoided at the time of EPD, although you may possibly tolerate a small amount of decaffeinated coffee.

Do not drink any kind of fruit juice until you are certain it will not cause you to have any adverse effects.

Extras

Hard margarine may be used as desired.

You can eat at least one serving of green vegetables every day. Small amounts of cabbage, Brussels sprouts, broccoli, cauliflower, or lettuce should be safe.

The mixed-flour cake and crispbread recipes may be eaten freely. Mixed flour can also be used for waffles and hot cakes.

Avoid these things at the time of EPD

As you may have noticed, this diet plan avoids many kinds of fruit including all citrus fruit. It also avoids butter, cheese, milk, and wheat products. It will be necessary for you expand your diet at some point. You may begin to add small amounts of these things when you are comfortable with the idea of experimenting and feel that you can do so successfully. Eat only small quantities at first.

More information about diet and EPD

If you are very sensitive to a particular food, you know that eating even the tiniest quantities can make you ill, but you can often avoid a reaction by eating a large amount of it at one time. In that way, you are masking its results. This masking effect lasts for five days and is part of the basis for the Four-Day Rotation Diet.

When you are part of the way through your EPD treatment, it becomes safe for you to eat small amounts of food you used to be able to eat safely only in a large, masking dose. At this time, since you may find that eating a large quantity of these foods will make you ill (unmasking), you may find it is necessary to change your diet.

When EPD is complete, you should be able to freely eat a normal, varied diet.

Alcohol

Alcoholic beverages contain low-molecular-weight extracts of food allergens and yeast, which are absorbed by the stomach extremely quickly. They may also contain corn, which is a strong allergen, as well as a wide variety of added chemicals.

Alcohol itself is known to be an immunosuppressant drug, but it may interfere with the effect of EPD even as late as the third week. Therefore, it is best to avoid alcohol completely during the first two weeks after EPD and be careful of its use afterward.

Coffee and tea

Many food-sensitive people believe that coffee and tea do not upset them, but both beverages contain important allergens that must be avoided at the time of EPD. Suddenly stopping the intake of coffee and tea can result in a severe withdrawal headache. To avoid this, it would be wise to reduce the consumption of tea and coffee gradually in the weeks preceding EPD treatment, perhaps switching to decaffeinated brands and stopping altogether several days before EPD. To protect against withdrawal, 50 mg tablets of caffeine may be taken once or twice daily. EPD is not affected by these.

Three important things to remember about diet and EPD

1. Rotation diets

   Rotating foods is not the same as mixing them. You should never use a rotating diet until at least two weeks after EPD, and then only if it is absolutely necessary. When EPD works, there is no longer any value in rotating your foods. Part way through a course of EPD, you may discover that your old rotating diet is likely to upset you. You can and should replace it with a more normal pattern of eating. It may be necessary to use the Very Mixed Diet during this change.

2. Introducing additional foods

   The full effect of a shot of EPD develops during the fourth

week. This is a time of transition. Before that time, you may become upset by eating foods that will be safe and comfortable for you to eat later on. You may experience a reaction to the dose during the first week or two. Do not assume that your symptoms are caused by your post-EPD diet.

3. Boosting tolerance

When EPD has been successful, you will be happy to discover you are able to eat as much as you want of any kind of food you want. Nevertheless, when you have another shot, you will have to go back to all the old restrictions so that the EPD can continue to boost your tolerance to the things that once upset you.

Since the doses of allergen contained in EPD are so small, the chance of a true acute generalized allergic reaction is extremely remote. However, it will be necessary for patients who receive the treatment by injection to remain under observation for thirty minutes or until the skin response to the treatment is obviously fading.

Delayed reactions to EPD are unpredictable and usually involve a temporary return of the allergies being treated. They should be controlled by medication or by avoidance of the offending allergen until the reaction passes. Delayed reactions may begin any time between two hours and five days after a shot of EPD. They may last a few days, occasionally two weeks, and very rarely, two months.

Delayed reactions may develop after any dose of EPD, but later doses will frequently cause no reaction. These reactions are to be taken as a good sign since they are usually followed by a favorable response to treatment. It is rare for the symptoms that are produced by such a reaction to require more treatment or to seem worse than the original illness.

Local reactions involve swelling around the site of treatment. They appear after three to six hours, rarely persist for longer than three days, and should obviously subside by the fourth day. After EPD injections, swellings can occasionally involve the entire forearm. If the cup technique has been used, swelling as large as the diameter of an egg may occur. This is common and is not a reason to remove the cup prematurely. They are associated with a good immunological response and should not necessarily be treated with any local treatment, although an antihistamine tablet may be used if severe discomfort persists.

Although it is extremely rare, it is possible for late infection after cup treatment to occur. When this happens, it is an allergic reaction in the scarification after the treatment is applied. Phagocytes migrate from the body into the cup, which then becomes filled with a thick, yellow, jellylike mass. When the cup is removed, the jelly should be allowed to dry because it will prevent bacteria from entering the scarification. It should not be swabbed with disinfectant.

After the third day, the area will be well protected by the healing scab. If it becomes hot or inflamed, there is an indication that bacteria have infected the wound. Furacin ointment or an antibiotic such as penicillin may be prescribed by the doctor.

Pigmentation after cup treatment can occur because the scarification is an unusual shallow injury to the skin. A faint bruise may remain after the skin has healed. This will fade slowly and may take months or even years to completely disappear. Mild sunburn can help the bruise disappear after the healed skin looks nearly normal.

In describing enzyme potentiated desensitization to other fellows and members of the American Association of Environmental Medicine in 1995, Dr. W.A. Shrader Jr., MD of the American EPD Society in Santa Fe, New Mexico, wrote: "If you knew of another method of therapy that doesn't involve permanent lifestyle changes, will likely end after a period of time, needs only be given every two months or less, and achieves a 70 percent success rate in the treatment of the chemically ill patient without having them have to live like hermits, I'd hope you'd want to share it with the rest of us. . . . I simply feel very strongly that the data now at hand clearly indicates that we owe the use of EPD to our patients." Enzyme potentiated desensitization is a method of therapy that will likely end after a period of time, needs only be given every two months or less, and achieves a 70 percent success rate in the treatment of the chemically ill without requiring a drastic change in lifestyle. In fact, other than local reactions at the injection site, there have been no serious side effects reported.

15

How to Live with
Multiple Chemical Sensitivity

IF YOUR CAR suddenly started to make strange noises, would you turn the radio up to disguise the rattling and thumping or would you take it to the mechanic to find out what was causing the noise? Of course you would take it to the mechanic and fix it before things got worse. When your car's alarms start to go off and the little red lights tell you that something is wrong, you know you have to deal with it right away.

The symptoms of multiple chemical sensitivity are suffering are your body's "alarms." They are trying to tell you that something is wrong. Although specific symptoms are your body's way of telling you what is harming you, it is up to you to listen carefully to what your body is saying. What should you do about these alarms? The important thing is to start looking for the origins of these signals. Ask yourself why your body is no longer functioning normally. Like your car, you have to find out what's wrong and fix it before it gets worse.

Certainly your doctor will temporarily treat your symptoms to relieve your pain, but if you are going to return to optimal health, you may have to accept the fact that your lifestyle is going to change. You must be willing to take charge of your life and of your personal world, to make serious accommodations and adjustments. A physician who is highly skilled in all aspects of environmental medicine can help you return to a reasonably normal way of life, but he can't do it all for you. Your doctor can be your advisor, coach, guide, even your cheerleader, but you are the only person who is available to change your surroundings twenty-four hours a day, seven days a week. When you can do that, you can help your body begin to heal itself.

Although there are some basic similarities, everyone's story is different because everyone's body is different and everyone's life is different. Your symptoms and the solutions for your problems can vary a great deal from somebody else's symptoms and solutions.

The one thing we all share is the unavoidable fact that toxicity presents a threat to a vibrant level of health. Whether you allow yourself to continue to be a victim of the adverse effects of toxicity depends on how much you know, how much you understand, and the choices you are willing to make to help yourself. This includes learning what is necessary to help your body protect itself. It also includes learning how to support your body's efforts to eliminate accumulated toxins. Unfortunately, by the time you become fully aware of what is causing your sickness, the "spreading phenomenon" may have already taken effect. You may have developed sensitivities to many additional items such as pollens, molds, and foods. You will possibly also have developed nutrient deficiencies. However, with the appropriate direction, you can take charge. You can make changes and you can help yourself.

You may find some changes troublesome and others burdensome. It won't be exactly the same free and easy lifestyle you enjoyed before you got sick. Many of the things you will be asked to do won't seem the least bit normal to you at first, but when you start to feel better you will agree that everything you are doing to help yourself is worth the inconvenience. It's important to understand why you are making these changes and how they are going to help you.

Detoxification

Detoxification involves actively working on the body to remove toxins, and detoxication involves the body's ability to remove toxins on its own. Both are extremely important. Equally important is finding a properly trained environmental physician who is willing to work with you to discover how, when, and why your sickness began, what caused it, and the degree to which it has progressed.

If your sickness is diagnosed in its early stages, it is possible that simply cleaning up your personal environment can go a long way toward easing your symptoms. Sometimes doing something as simple as improving ventilation and regularly replacing furnace and air conditioning filters can help. If you have become acutely toxic, however, you will have no choice but to stay away from any type of exposure until you are completely detoxified.

The two names to remember in the detoxification game are nutrition and avoidance. Avoiding those things that potentially cause you to suffer from chemical stress can decrease your body's total burden by allowing your own overtaxed detoxication systems to recover. It may be necessary for you to start out by avoiding specific places and things. It may even be necessary to avoid certain people because of the cosmetics and toiletries they regularly use.

Toxic materials can include stored or leaking chemicals, dyes, gasoline, paints, solvents, glues, acids, insecticides, or cleaning agents among others. If you are aware of the sources of toxic materials at home or at work, remove as many of them as you can. If it is not possible for you to remove or avoid these materials, at least wear protective clothing and a breathing apparatus when you must come into contact with them.

A less toxic environment and a healthy detoxication system are required to repair your health. The unfortunate fact is that severely affected people will have no choice but to leave badly polluted areas. Changing your job may be the only way you can restore your health. You may be forced to abandon the surroundings of a large city so that you can live on a mountain or at the seashore.

Water and juice fasts were once the preferred methods of detoxication. They were believed to work on the principle that, once the body was relieved of the "stress" of digestion and the further accumulation of toxins was eliminated, it would be able to clear stored toxins and heal itself. Further research has shown that that the body's detoxication mechanism involves a heavily nutrient-supported process. Protein losses caused by prolonged water and juice fasts can actually weaken muscles and organs, which can cause a gradual slowing of metabolic activity as the body tries to conserve its depleted energy resources.

So, simple juice or water fasting is no longer a desirable method of detoxification. The better approach involves thoroughly nourishing the body so that its natural detoxication mechanisms are fueled by the nutrients needed to achieve the highest level of detoxication activity. By providing high quality protein, complex carbohydrates, and essential fats, the body can prevent muscle and organ breakdown and avoid depleted energy resources. Nutrients are needed to support the function of those organs directly involved in detoxication. These include the liver, the intestinal tract, the skin, and the kidneys.

Your doctor will design a personal detoxification program for you. This will probably include a daily routine of balanced meals, regular rest, and the avoidance of drugs, alcohol, and medications, combined with appropriate exercise. It may include aerobic exercise and a low-temperature sauna for a short time after exercise to stimulate the excretion of toxic substances through the skin. Water, salt, and potassium replacements and nutritional supplements may be administered orally and intravenously. There will be calcium and magnesium supplements and the use of polyunsaturated oils to help remove toxins from the intestine. Injection therapy may be used for inhalants, foods, and some chemicals. It might also be important to spend time in a biodetoxification center, where heat therapy can be much more aggresive uner medical supervision.

If you are overweight, weight reduction and management is important, since fat is an important factor in dealing with multiple chemical sensitivity. Fat provides a storage site that is ready and waiting to accept and hold the fat-loving toxins. Once they are deposited in the fat, toxins are particularly difficult to remove. Unless the excess fat is removed, these harmful chemicals remain in your body, continuing to be a source of toxicity. To understand how important this is, a chemical like DDT has a half-life of fifteen to twenty years when stored in the fat deposits of the body.

Food

People once appreciated good food for the value of its nutrition and for the pleasure it provided. In recent times, food has come to be perceived as a threat, a source of guilt, a dangerous substance filled with unnatural products. By eating wholesome, nutritious foods, your food can again become a source of nutrition and pleasure.

Nutrition is an important step on the road to health. A sound diet including plenty of fresh, wholesome foods avoids processed foods and foods in which chemicals are routinely used as additives, preservatives, or ripening agents. Avoid foods that contain hormones and antibiotics used in production. Whenever possible, use organically raised meat and organically grown fruits and vegetables.

Do you really know where your next meal is coming from? The fruit in your fresh fruit salad plate may have traveled all the way from Peru, the Middle East, or China. Produce may be hauled from one side of the continent to the other, or even from one side of the world to the other, before it is treated, stored, and distributed. It may have been treated with all kinds of pesticides, some of which are no longer acceptable for use by this nation. It may have been picked while it was still green then treated with gases to force the unripe food to ripen. Or it may have been injected with artificial food coloring to make it look like the "real thing."

Why would you want to put this artificial stuff into your body when you can buy fresh food? Organically grown natural foods have up to 50 percent more nutritive value than commonly available, generically produced, commercially grown products.

Fresh food not only helps you improve your health, it also tastes better. If you have never eaten a fresh home-grown tomato, you don't know what a tomato tastes like. Fresh asparagus doesn't taste like that gray stuff you find in a can, and freshly harvested potatoes are so flavorful you don't need added butter or salt. It is unfortunate that the special requirements and limited market cause organically grown fruits and vegetables to be more expensive than the mass produced variety, but when you consider the costs, they're not nearly as expensive as staying sick.

Some inconvenience may be involved in eating only fresh, naturally grown foods. Every kind of produce will not be available to you all the time. You won't be able to get strawberries and peaches in the middle of winter. You may not find rutabagas in the summer. Our grandparents knew that fresh fruits and vegetables are not only seasonal, they are also fragile. Organically grown fruits and vegetables are not treated with the preservatives that cause commercial foods to seem to last forever. Every zucchini and banana comes with its own built-in time clock. You can no longer expect to shop today and eat the produce you buy two weeks from now. You will be obliged to shop more often and pay a premium for what you purchase. You will find yourself purchasing fewer things and using them quickly before they spoil. You will also find yourself enjoying fresher, tastier, and more nutritious food.

Find your local farmers market or locate a farmer who grows produce by organic methods. If this isn't possible, find an organic or whole foods store where you can buy fresh vegetables that are guaranteed to have been grown without additional chemicals. Find a butcher who can provide free-range fowl and cattle that is grown without hormones or antibiotics.

Years ago people did their own canning and preserving. Cakes, pies, puddings, sauces, soups, and condiments were made at home where the family cook knew exactly what was put in them. Now we now find ourselves tempted by a bewildering array of ready-made, preprocessed, packaged, canned, and preserved foods. Some of these may be labeled "health" food, "organic," "nonorganic," or "nonallergenic" food. In spite of these fancy labels, there is no universally safe food. You must read product labels carefully and search for those foods allowed on your specific diet. Commercially prepared foods are quick to use and easy to prepare, but even after reading the labels carefully, many of their ingredients are indecipherable and they lack much of the nutrition we are seeking.

It is possible to create your own convenience foods by freezing, canning, or drying them at home. Prepare several meals at one time and freeze them for later use. You can package vegetables separately for freezing. Freeze fruit and vegetable juice in ice cube trays for later use, and use a hydrator to prepare dried foods. Consult a home economist, county agent, or public library to learn about safe home canning techniques.

You will also learn to change your cooking methods. You will choose to avoid foods that are grilled, fried, barbecued, or roasted since carcinogenic compounds are created by heat damage to fats and protein. Instead, use slow baking or wok cooking at 320 degrees Fahrenheit. It is better to use the microwave only when absolutely necessary to reheat foods.

Avoid eating excess fat and refined sugar. Eat moderate levels of protein while increasing levels of complex carbohydrates.

People who take frequent antibiotics, use multiple drugs, eat a lot of sweets, and have low nutrient levels crucial to the detoxication system are most likely to become affected by a toxic environment. Once these deficiencies are discovered, the integrity of the detoxication system can be restored. A healthful diet that is high in nutrients can help your body with the detoxication process. Vitamin and mineral supplements are often necessary to replace deficiencies resulting from direct toxic damage.

Failure to reduce the total body load before pollutant challenge will frequently yield inaccurate results. It is essential to conduct investigative procedures in controlled environmental circumstances with the total load reduced. Your doctor or her dietitian will provide a diet program specifically designed for your needs.

Rotary diet

A rotary diet of less chemically contaminated food may be required to reduce your body's load and keep you in the unmasked state. It must be noted that, as helpful as it is, the rotary diet doesn't work for everyone. For this reason, it should be advised and monitored carefully by your environmental physician. If your environmental physician finds that this diet is not working for you, he will recommend one of the many other available programs. A properly balanced rotary diet can be important in discovering and treating food sensitivities. Since the rotary diet only allows you to eat a specific food once during a set time, the rotation prevents the food from becoming still another sensitizing agent. The rotary diet has many nutritional advantages. It is high in fiber and low in salt because it uses whole, less refined foods.

Since a food usually remains in your body three to four days or longer, an offending food is most likely to produce symptoms if a second meal of it is eaten before the first meal leaves your body. On the rotary diet nothing you eat, whether it be food, beverages, or seasonings, may be eaten more often than once every four to seven days or more.

Eight principles of a rotary diet

1. Omit all junk food such as candies, cakes, pies cookies, soft drinks, and processed and prepared foods containing additives, preservatives, and food coloring.

2. No food is to be eaten more often than once every four days. For example, a food eaten on Monday may not be eaten again until Friday.

3. Canned fruits and vegetables are discouraged.

4. Foods may be eaten raw or cooked by steaming, boiling, broiling, baking, or frying in its own fat.

5. Drink and cook with spring water in glass containers.

6. Rotate herbal teas as alternatives to daily coffee and tea.

7. Be sure all meals are three to four hours apart.

8. Do not eat longer than one hour at each meal.

Four days of the rotary diversified diet

Day 1
Protein: Chicken, Cornish hen, turkey, goose, duck, rabbit, squirrel, tuna, mackerel, sea bass, grouper

Vegetables: Broccoli, cabbage, cauliflower, brussels sprouts, water chestnuts, breadfruit

Fruits: Banana, strawberry, raspberry, blackberry, pineapple, guava

Starch or Grain: Breadfruit, sweet potato, agar agar

Seeds and Nuts: Walnuts, pecans, macadamia nuts, lichee nuts

Sweetener: Cocoa, honey, vanilla, pineapple

Spice and Seasoning: Basil, oregano, sage, rosemary, thyme, mustard seed, horseradish

Oils and Fats: Chicken, duck, turkey, flax seed oil

Beverages and Teas: Guava juice, pineapple juice, raspberry juice, spearmint tea

Day 2

Protein: (All red meats and their byproducts) Beef, veal, lamb, goat, buffalo, pork, milk, cheese, yogurt, sardines, herring, red snapper

Vegetables: Potato, green pepper, onion, asparagus, garlic, lettuce, artichoke, olives, mushrooms

Fruits: Apple, pear, avocado, grape, raisin, peach, cherry, apricot, plum, prickly pear, mango, tomato

Starch or Grain: rice, oat, millet, wheat, barley, wild rice, sunflower meal, potato

Seeds and Nuts: Cashew, pistachio, filbert, chestnut, hazelnut, almonds, sunflower seeds

Sweetener: Almond syrup, rice syrup, cane sugar, malt syrup, grape concentrate

Spice and Seasoning: Allspice, cloves, bay leaves, cinnamon, paprika, chives, onion

Oils and Fats: Butter, lard, olive oil, almond, apricot oil, safflower oil

Beverages and Teas: Apple juice, milk, tomato juice, goat milk, grape juice, chamomile tea

Day 3

Protein: (Shellfish) Crab, shrimp, lobster, trout, salmon, abalone, clams, oysters, scallops, swordfish

Vegetables: Carrot, celery, parsnip, squash, cucumber, zucchini, pumpkin, okra

Fruits: Cantaloupe, honeydew, other melons, persimmon, rhubarb, pomegranate, kiwi fruit

Starch or Grain: Buckwheat, amaranth, quinoa, sesame meal, lotus root

Seeds and Nuts: Pumpkin seeds, sesame seeds, pine nuts

Sweetener: Maple sugar, syrup and granules, persimmon

Spice and Seasoning: Dill, parsley, caraway, anise, fennel, coriander

Oils and Fats: Sesame oil, cottonseed oil, pumpkin oil

Beverages and Teas: Carrot juice, pomegranate juice, watermelon juice

DAY 4

Protein: (Fish) Halibut, sole, turbot, catfish, cod, haddock, pike

Vegetables: All peas, beans, and sprouts; jicama; spinach; beets; yams

Fruits: Blueberry, cranberry, orange, lime, lemon, grapefruit, dates, coconut, papaya

Starch or Grain: Arrowroot, tapioca, cassava, malanga, mung and green beans, noodles, yucca

Seeds and Nuts: Peanuts, soy nuts, brazil nuts, chestnuts

Sweetener: Date sugar, coconut, carob, beet sugar

Spice and Seasonings: Nutmeg, mace, lemon, black and white pepper

Oils and Fats: Coconut oil, peanut oil, soy oil, fish oil

Beverages and Teas: Lemonade, orange juice, coconut milk, papaya juice, cranberry juice

Alternative foods for the rotary diet:

FLOURS:

Amaranth, arrowroot, Jerusalem artichoke, plantain, buckwheat, cassava, chickpea, lima bean, lotus root, malanga, nut and seed flours, oats, peanuts, potato, quinoa, rice, sesame, soybean, tapioca, water chestnut, white sweet potato, yam

Egg Alternatives:
Arrowroot mixture, baking powder mixture, dried fruit puree, egg replacer, flaxseed mixture, soybean curd

Oils:
Almond, apricot kernel, avocado, beef drippings, chicken fat, coconut, cottonseed, olive, peanut, palm kernel, pumpkin, safflower, sesame, soy, sunflower

Milk Substitutes:
Almond meal, banana milk, coconut milk, goat's milk, nut or seed milk, pineapple juice, potato milk, soy milk, special foods milk (cassava, lotus root, malanga, water chestnut, white sweet potato), vegetable juices, zucchini milk

Sweeteners:
Aquamiel, almond syrup, carob, date sugar, dried fruit, fig concentrate, honey, licorice sweetener, malt (barley), maple syrup, rice syrup, (cautious use of beet, cane, and corn sugars)

Leavenings:
Baking soda, baking powder recipe, special foods baking powder

Cereals and Meals:
Amaranth (puffed and cereal), buckwheat (cereal and flakes), crispy cereal shreds; special foods (malanga, cassava, yam, etc.), millet flakes, rice (cereal and puffed), special foods creamed cereals (lotus root, amaranth, etc.), quinoa (puffed and cereal)

Pastas and Noodles:
Buckwheat, bifun (rice and potato), green bean noodles, saifun

(sweet potato starch), kuzikuri, mung bean noodles, special foods pasta (amaranth, cassava, yam, etc.)

VEGETABLE AND FRUIT CHIPS:
Artichoke chips, banana rice petals, carrot chips, cassava chips, malanga chips, parsnip chips, potato chips, plantain chips, sweet potato chips

CRACKERS:
Amaranth, cassava, brown rice, lotus root, malanga, white sweet potato, yam

Walter

Even though the United States has one of the best water supply systems in the world, recent outbreaks of waterborne illnesses in places like Las Vegas, Washington, and Milwaukee have demonstrated that our water supply may be less than perfect. If you are chemically sensitive, you may decide to use less chemically contaminated water, including spring and charcoal-filtered water. Be sure to use only glass or steel containers. Although the hard polycarbonate plastics are probably safe, water can leach a variety of contaminants from the walls of some synthetic plastic containers.

A home water purification system is highly desirable to provide pure water for drinking and cooking. By all means, you will want to install a home water treatment system for your drinking water supply. Unfortunately, there are no federal, state, or local regulations that govern the manufacture or use of home water treatment systems, and you will find a confusing array of brands and types available at widely varying prices, ranging from a low-cost, carbon-activated carafe sink filter to an expensive and complex reverse osmosis system.

No single system can remove every possible contaminant from your water supply. No matter how expensive it is, how top of the line, state of the art it is, no product is capable of doing everything.

Each type of system involves different treatment technologies, and various treatment technologies are effective in removing different classes of contaminants. It would be a good idea to have your drinking water analyzed so that you will know what specific contaminants you need to remove before you purchase a filtration system. Some filtering systems will remove inorganics like sulfur or chlorine. Others do a good job of removing lead but won't remove pathogens. The very best combination is a carbon and reversed osmosis system.

After you decide which system you require and you install it or have it installed, you will have to commit your time and energy to a dedicated program of maintenance, changing filters, and monitoring of performance on a regular schedule. If you don't change filters regularly or service your system regularly, harmful contaminants may build up so that you may wind up drinking worse water than you started with. Some systems require changing the filters every two months or after using thirty-five gallons of water. Some systems automatically shut off when the filter's time has expired.

The reverse osmosis system is both expensive and possibly the most effective home purification system available. Pressurized water is forced across semipermeable membranes. The purified water is then passed through another filter and stored in a pressurized tank. Lead, arsenic, and certain pathogens are filtered out by the system, but 50 to 90 percent of the water that goes through the system is discarded.

Activated carbon filtration systems are among the simplest systems available. Water pours through solid block carbon filters. These may be as simple as the carbon-activated carafe filter that attaches to your faucet or one of the more complex systems mounted on countertops or under the sink. Carbon-activated systems are effective in reducing lead contamination, chlorine, and sediment.

Distillation systems boil water, capture the steam, then recondense the vapor into drinking water. During the process most inorganic contaminants like lead will be removed and bacteria and pathogens will be killed, but it does little to remove such volatile chemicals as benzene.

Whichever system you select, you will need to drink plenty of purified water. Drink eight eight-ounce glasses of water every day.

Oasis

Regardless of our state of health, we all need a private place where we can find refuge from the world and all its problems. If you are chemically sensitive, your private place will be more than a retreat. It will be your haven from the chemical world that threatens your well-being. It will become your sheltering oasis, the one place where you are protected from the raging desert of chemical assaults. Properly outfitted, your oasis will become the safe haven to which you can escape after you have been chemically exposed.

At first, you will want to spend both day and night inside your oasis, to eat there and to sleep there in secure comfort. This can be considered rest time for your body. Your oasis may make it possible to relieve your symptoms without using medications. Free of chemical exposures, your immune system can recover from chemical susceptibility.

When you emerge from your filtered oasis after having spent several days and nights inside, you may find that you are sharply aware of the harmful and unpleasant fumes of certain chemicals. Some people can even taste chemical fumes. When that happens, you may immediately experience the return of your symptoms, or you may experience a delayed return of your symptoms. Since everyone responds differently to different incitants, your reaction will depend on many factors, including your particular chemical load and your state at the time of exposure. The important thing is that you do not allow yourself to become discouraged. In time your symptoms will be relieved more rapidly each time you return to the oasis. This is a good sign that your treatment is working, that the oasis is helping, and that your immune system is rebuilding itself.

The ideal location for your "oasis" would include a bedroom and bath combination. If this combination is not available at your house, choose a room with a door that can be kept closed, and if necessary, a towel can be placed across the threshold to protect you from outside fumes. Have someone else clean the oasis thoroughly and set it up to the proper specifications.

Perhaps the most important item in your oasis is the air filter. Get the best you can afford. It should be allowed to run constantly.

Heating should be provided by radiant electric heaters or hot water electric heaters.

Remove all furniture, draperies, and clothing from the room. If possible, remove all carpeting. If carpeting cannot be removed, remember that it is easier to tolerate nylon than polyesters. It is best to use washable cotton rugs or bare floors.

If the flooring is plywood, it would be a good idea to cover it with a barrier cloth or mylar "space blanket" because plywood is glued together with petrochemical glues and resins. If the flooring is vinyl, cover it with barrier cloth unless it is old and the odors have already been completely released. Ceramic tile floors are best, particularly if the grout is old. Wash the floors thoroughly with borax or baking soda and water.

Although you would like your oasis to be clean and fresh, this is definitely not the time to repaint the walls. Instead, clean the walls by washing them either with borax or with a combination of baking soda and water. Do not use a room that has vinyl wallpaper or wallpaper that was applied with adhesives containing insecticides. Unsealed pine surfaces should be covered with barrier cloth.

If it is necessary for privacy, your windows may be covered with washable cotton curtains. Organic cotton sheets can be used to make practical, washable, and attractive draperies.

Every bit of clothing should be removed from the room's closet. While you are in your oasis, wear only cotton clothing and store only cotton clothing in the closets. Do not allow polyester or polyester blend clothing to remain in the room. No woolen or dry cleaned articles should be allowed to remain in the room because the formaldehyde cleaning solution lingers on the clothing. When all these precautions have been taken, it is time to return only those furnishings that are absolutely necessary for comfort and daily use. Limit the furnishings. In furnishing the oasis, it is best to imagine that you are discarding a plush, cluttered, overstuffed Victorian ambiance in favor of one that is more nearly contemporary, scaled down, uncluttered, and clean lined.

Select a bed frame that is all metal or wood and be sure that it has been thoroughly cleaned with borax or baking soda and water. Or, if necessary, the mattress can be placed directly on the floor. The mattress, pillows, and box springs should not contain sponge rubber, urethane foam, or any other synthetic fabrics. The best choice is a 100 percent organic cotton mattress. Several varieties are available. If you cannot replace your mattress, enclose the mattress and box springs with a space blanket that is sealed at the seams or with one of the new mattress coverings available for this purpose.

Do not use blankets or sheets made of synthetic fabrics. Use 100 percent cotton materials that have not been treated to be "permanent press." White or natural fabrics are best because the dyes in colored or printed sheets may have offensive odors.

If possible, bed pillows should also be 100 percent organic cotton covered with 100 percent cotton pillowcases. If cotton pillows are not available, place several folded cotton towels in a pillowcase. Freshly laundered down or feather pillows are acceptable for use by those people who are not sensitive to feathers.

A table or desk should be made of wood, glass, or metal. If plastic TV tables are brought into the oasis, test for reactions if symptoms are at base line.

Use wooden chairs. Soften them with cotton-filled, washable fabric chair pads. If your only available chairs are upholstered with vinyl, the vinyl area should be covered with barrier cloth and sealed.

Lamps with ceramic, glass, or wooden bases are best. Do not use plastic lamp bases or plastic shades that can give off odors when they heat. Clean lamps thoroughly with borax or baking soda and water.

You may have a hard plastic clock and a hard plastic radio and tape player. It would be advisable to run a new TV set outside your oasis for several days to allow odors to be released. Remember to move all these appliances from the oasis before retiring for the night. The telephone can become a problem because, after a while, you may be able to smell or even taste its plastic fumes. Cover the mouthpiece with a clean cotton sock. This telephone "slipcover" should prevent discomfort.

As you begin to be more comfortable in your oasis, it is perfectly natural that you will want to experiment with more furnishings and add more of your normal comforts. Be careful not to bring in new items into the oasis without testing them. The most reasonable way to do this is to introduce one new item at a time. When you are sure you can tolerate that item, you may introduce another.

If you are sensitive to newsprint, read the newspaper only in a book box. Dust papers and books with baking soda to reduce acidic fumes.

If it is necessary for you to use a typewriter while you are in your oasis, remember not to type for long periods of time. Inks in the ribbon and film can provoke chemical stress. Of course you will want to remove the typewriter before you go to bed at night. The same restrictions should apply to you computer, printer, scanner, fax machine, and related equipment.

Do not accumulate books, papers, and newspapers inside the oasis. Store them somewhere else.

You will not keep cosmetics, perfumes, aftershave lotions, scented powders, or toiletries in the oasis, and it is important to remind friends and family members not to use these items when they visit.

Even though smokers may be considerate enough to smoke out of doors or even outside the house altogether, the odors of tobacco smoke remain in their clothing, on their skin, and in their hair. You can't afford to be kind or generous or loving. Smokers and the odors they bring with them simply cannot be welcomed into your oasis. If you live with a family of artists, sculptors, farmers, house painters, printers, or chemical workers, have them remain outside the oasis until they have showered and changed clothing. Their work clothes should be washed as soon as they are finished with them.

When your symptoms improve, you will be able to spend an increasingly longer time outside the oasis. Eventually you will be able to return to the outside world for the greatest part of your day, perhaps only retreating to your oasis at night or to recover after you have suffered a chemical insult.

Home Environment

As you spend more time outside your oasis, it will become necessary to clean up your home to create a safe environment. Although the rest of your house may not have to be as Spartan as the inside of your oasis, this is going to involve the most drastic and traumatic spring cleaning you have ever undertaken in your life. It will be considerably more complicated than merely dusting under the beds and washing the windows.

Start at one end of the house and work your way to the other end. Your goal is to reach a symptom-free base line for other parts of your home outside your oasis. Once a symptom-free base line is reached, you will have achieved an "ecologically safe" home.

To do this, you will have to isolate home exposures so that you can avoid them or remove them. If you suspect an item such as carpeting, put a fair amount of it in a closed room that is free of other fumes. Leave it there for a week. After a week you can test yourself by sitting in the room for as long as thirty minutes. If symptoms occur, that item must be removed.

As home exposures are isolated one by one, you will remove as many household incitants as possible, including petroleum-derived heat sources, insecticides, synthetic carpets and mattresses, and formaldehyde-containing substances such as pressboard and plywood.

If you are susceptible to natural gas, consider removing your gas oven and range for a week as you watch for symptoms. If your symptoms improve considerably when the gas appliances are gone, by all means replace them with electric appliances.

If you have an attached garage, keep the door to the garage closed. Seal it if you can or use it only when absolutely necessary.

Remove highly odorous materials such as chlorine bleaches and cleansers, ammonia, detergents, disinfectants, solvents, dry cleaning materials and lighter fluids, paint, varnish, turpentine, and mineral spirits.

Avoid room deodorants, potpourri, scented fabric softeners, scented washing products, perfumes, colognes, scented hair spray, mousse or shampoo, scented soaps, and cosmetics. Although deodorizers make your house smell springtime fresh, the real purpose of most deodorizers and air fresheners is to desensitize your nose so that you are no longer offended by those offensive indoor odors. They use cresol, phenol, and formaldehyde, which are responsible for many health problems. Although houseplants can absorb pollutants and purify the air, they can also become moldy. If so, they can create problems for some people who are suffering from multiple chemical sensitivity. Baking soda is a harmless natural alternative. Baking soda or white vinegar may be placed around the house in small dishes. Baking soda will absorb odors in the refrigerator, trash cans, and kitty litter pans. If there is a bad smell inside your house, clean it up or open the window to let it out. Check your kitchen, pantry, bathroom, closets, drawers, and cabinets to find the source of strong or offensive odors and get rid of them.

Avoid using insecticides and repellents, mothballs, chlordane, and parathion. To prevent moths from nibbling up your clothes, fold cedar blocks in clean woolens or store woolens in cedar chests or closets. Cedar balls are effective and can be renewed with sandpaper. A gauze bag containing cedar chips can be decorative as well as effective. Or you can discourage moths with a sweet-scented pomander, using two handfuls each of dried lavender and rosemary plus one tablespoon each of fresh cloves and dried lemon peel secured in a gauze bag.

Remember, if house and garden pesticides are strong enough to kill the bugs, large doses are not going to do you any good. Pesticides contain some of the most toxic synthetic chemicals ever developed. They have been linked to birth defects, leukemia, and cancer. Pesticides are long lasting and find their way into the water supply, killing fish and wildlife and contaminating our drinking waters. Creative alternatives in the garden may include introducing beneficial bugs to attack pests, using organic insecticides and fertilizers, and simple companion planting. Insect traps may be used in the home. Biological pesticides use species-specific bacteria to kill pests.

Of course, you will not allow tobacco smoke anywhere inside your home. This is easier to do than you think. Hide all your decorative ash trays and just say no. These days smokers are accustomed to taking their habit outside in all kinds of weather.

Pollens can be a significant irritant so avoid exposure to pollens, especially at the height of the pollen season when you may need to limit your outdoor activity. Whenever possible, stay inside and use an air purifier. You may even find that wearing a special face mask is helpful.

Nobody is going to tell you to part with your beloved pet, but if you don't own a pet before you are diagnosed with multiple chemical sensitivity, don't get one. No matter how much you love your pet and no matter how much he loves you, you have to keep him out of your bedroom. Don't let him sleep on your bed. Clean the areas the pet uses thoroughly and often. Weekly shampooing and conditioning not only reduces the risk of fleas and ticks, it also removes dander and other irritants.

Mold can be a major problem if you live in a heavily wooded area or if you live near the beach, lakes, rivers, or streams. Outdoor plantings can contribute to mold formation inside the house. It may be necessary to remove shrubs or to prune plants close to your house. Houseplants can also contribute to mold problems. Mold may grow in potting soil and stems. Crushed rock on top of the soil around each plant can add a decorative effect and reduce the number of mold spores in the air. In summer you can keep houseplants outdoors.

Molds thrive in cool, damp, and poorly ventilated areas including basements, bathrooms, refrigerators, garbage pails, and those dark places under the sink. Use borax or zephrin and clean all your mold-prone areas often. Use nontoxic cleaning agents like borax or zephrin to clean air conditioners, humidifiers, dehumidifiers, and vaporizers and keep them free of mold. Check behind wallpaper and paneling and under carpets or carpet pads for mold.

Throw away all those old magazines and newspapers you have collected, and dust or vacuum your books frequently.

No matter where you are in your house or at work, avoid as many unnecessary commercial cleaning products as possible.

Bathrooms

Molds grow in bathroom drains, on damp towels, on washcloths, in shower stalls, and in every possible crevice. Use an exhaust fan to circulate the air and keep the bathroom dry. Since mold thrives in the warm, wet atmosphere that is found in most bathrooms, check corner areas and areas under the sink and behind the commode for mold growth. Scrub grout, tiles, and bathroom appliances with disinfectant. Don't leave damp towels or clothing in the hamper. Avoid using unnecessary decorative accessories in the bathroom. Use cotton bath-mats and clean them often.

Mold and mildew cleaners contain pesticides that can cause eye and skin irritation or lung damage. A simple solution of Borax and water or vinegar and water will clean problem areas. Borax will inhibit the growth of molds. To prevent the return of mold and mildew, keep the area clean and well ventilated.

Don't allow shower curtains to remain bunched up or to stick to the wall or the tub where it can mildew.

If you have a clothes hamper in the bathroom, don't let it fill with damp, soiled clothing. Widely used by careful people to poison germs in the home, most disinfectants contain a poisonous brew of phenol, formaldehyde, cresol, ammonia, or chlorine. A mixture of 1/2 cup borax to one gallon of hot water is a safe, convenient germicide.

Commercial toilet bowl cleaners do their job well, but most of the time they do it with chlorine or hypochorous acid, which can burn your skin and harm your eyes. The fumes alone can corrode metal. When a manufacturer's warning label tells you not to breath the product you are using, don't use it. Instead, use soap and borax to clean and disinfect. To remove stubborn rings, pour 1/2 cup vinegar into the toilet and let it sit for up to an hour before rinsing.

Basements

If your basement is damp, dry it out. Seal any cracks in the walls or floors, and use a dehumidifier. Increased ventilation and lighting discourage the growth of mold. Discard unused or unuseable stored items.

Bedrooms

Since you spend approximately a third of your life in your bedroom, it should get your special attention. Although it might not be as strictly prepared as your oasis, it should receive some special care. Use a cotton barrier cloth cover on your mattress. Do not use plastic covers. The chemical odors can be harmful. Select your bedding carefully. Use natural fabrics such as linen or cotton sheets and pillowcases. You won't want to use chenille bedspreads or fuzzy blankets. Clean mattresses and bed clothes frequently, and don't store anything under your bed.

Remove all carpets and rugs. They give off chemical fumes, and they capture and hold dust and molds. Use cotton mats in cold weather.

Avoid wall hangings, stuffed toys, and other dust catchers. Remove heavy draperies and curtains. Use shades, washable cotton curtains, or aluminum blinds instead.

Remove heavily stuffed furniture. Wooden chairs and furniture are safest.

Change air duct filters regularly and use a filter or damp cheesecloth over vents to reduce the circulation of dust. Heat your bedroom with an electric heater and use a separate window air conditioner. Use an air purifier for this room. Keep all doors and windows closed.

Keep all clothing in closed closets or drawers, never lying about the room. It may even be necessary to remove clothing storage from the bedroom area.

Living Areas

Avoid carpets, heavy draperies, and heavily stuffed furniture. Avoid any furniture that is upholstered with synthetic textiles, dacron, orlon, polyester, or rayon, as well as furniture that is stuffed with feathers or down.

Keep books in closed bookcases. They are notorious for collecting mold, dust, and dust mites. Clean and vacuum regularly. It is possible to get a vacuum that does not throw dust back into the house.

Use air purifiers and filters. Check humidifiers, air conditioners, and vaporizers constantly and clean them frequently.

Avoid using pine- or cedar-scented furniture polish. Wood floor and furniture polishes often contain phenol, which causes cancer in animals. As little as one thimbleful of phenol can cause circulatory collapse, even death. Worse, residual vapors remain in the home long after application. Wood polish may cause severe skin irritation. Keep your wood furniture dusted. Wipe occasionally with a barely damp cloth and polish finished wood with butcher's wax once or twice a year.

Solvents and fungicides are among the most toxic substances found in commercial oil and latex paints. Harmful vapors can be emitted for months after the paint dries. When you are painting, always be sure to protect yourself with gloves and a face mask. Use nontoxic vegetable-based paints, stains, and lacquers, or finish woods with natural wax finishes.

Glass cleaning products contain either ammonia or chlorine, and when you mist the windows and mirrors, you breathe ammonia or chlorine mist. Worse, they leave residual wax on the surface to trap dirt and dust. Use rubbing alcohol to remove the residual wax, then clean glass with a mixture of 1/2 white vinegar and 1/2 water.

Dining Room

Avoid plastic cutlery, drinking cups, and dinnerware. Set your table with china, porcelain, ceramics, and glass. Avoid plastic table covers, place mats, and chair pads. Whenever possible, use cotton, which can be laundered frequently.

Kitchen

As with the bathroom, molds love your kitchen drains, towels, and sponges. Keep your kitchen clean and dry. If the inside of your refrigerator looks as though it is growing science fair projects, clean it out and keep it clean. Use a nontoxic cleaning agent to scrub refrigerator shelves and doors. Don't store small bits of cooked food until they are unuseable. Dispose of them.

Don't use soft plastics. Instead, use natural materials like ceramic, glass, or wood for bowls and storage. Use cellophane bags instead of plastic. Keep all trash containers emptied and clean.

Drain cleaners are among the most dangerous products to be found in the home. They use lye and hydrochloric or sulfuric acids, which can burn human tissue and cause permanent damage. If not used precisely according to instructions, they can explode! To keep drains clean, make a solution of 1/2 cup baking soda, 1/2 cup salt, and 1/8 cup cream of tartar. Pour this mixture down the drain and follow it with hot water. Since the mixture does not remain effective if stored, it is best to mix only as much as needed. If a drain is clogged, pour 1/4 cup of baking soda down the drain, and follow it with 1/2 cup vinegar. There will be an immediate fizzing. Cover the drain until the fizzing stops, then flush it with hot water. And of course, always use a drain basket to prevent problems before they start.

Use a nontoxic cleaning agent to keep work surfaces, cutting boards, and cabinets clean. Although isobutane, propane, and butane used in popular aerosol products don't destroy the earth's ozone shield as many earlier aerosols did, animal studies indicate they may be toxic to the heart and central nervous system. When a spray is absolutely necessary, pump dispensers are efficient and easy to use.

Many common all-purpose cleaning products contain either ammonia or chlorine. Ammonia is harmful to the lungs, and chlorine can produce cancer-causing compounds. Every homemaker knows or should know that when products containing both ammonia and chlorine are mixed together they form a deadly chloramine gas. It would be better to clean with hot water, soap, and borax. Or use 1/2 cup washing soda dissolved in a bucket of water for all-purpose cleaning. This works for all but aluminum surfaces.

Dishwashing liquids smell nice and make a lot of bubbles, but most are detergents made from petroleum. Artificial fragrances and colors often give them the appearance of lemon or berry. Detergents cause more child poisoning than any other products. Liquid castile soap or naturally derived or glycerin-based soaps and a damp washcloth will get dishes equally clean.

Automatic dishwashing products contain strong detergents with high concentrations of phosphates they remain in the water stream, eventually killing fish and aquatic life. A solution of 50 percent borax and 50 percent washing soda works well in soft water and can be adjusted for use in harder water. If necessary, select the lowest phosphate detergent available and cut it with as much as 50 percent baking soda.

Vent the clothes dryer to the outside to help prevent the condensation of moisture, which can lead to the growth of mold.

Lye is the basic ingredient in oven cleaners. It is a powerful caustic that will blind you if you splash it in your eye, burn you if you get it on your skin, and scar your lungs if you inhale it. You don't want this stuff in the house, but you don't want a dirty oven either. Avoid spills and grease build up by lining the oven floor with aluminum foil. Clean the oven with a paste of baking soda and hot water. Use steel wool to remove difficult spots. Self-cleaning or continuous-cleaning ovens bypass the problem altogether.

Many of the popular laundry products are nonbiodegradable detergents made from petroleum products. It would be better to use soap products and boost them with washing soda and borax. Borax brightens washable fabrics, removes odors, and is more economical than bleach.

Sulfuric acids, phosphoric acids, and ammonia fumes from metal polishes contaminate the air inside the home. Silver flatware may be polished by lining a pan with heavyweight aluminum foil. Make a solution of equal parts of baking powder and salt. Fill the pan with warm water and soak the silver flatware until tarnish disappears.

To clean copper, mix lemon juice with hot vinegar and salt. To clean aluminum, dip a cloth in lemon juice, polish, then rinse with warm water.

Your Car

Your automobile has the potential for becoming a dangerous place for you to be, but our mobile lifestyles make it impossible to avoid driving from one place to another. With some thought and care, it can become as safe and comfortable as your home.

It is best to keep the car windows closed to keep as much incitant-laden air out of the car as possible. Use the car's air conditioner to recirculate the air in order to reduce the amount of outside air that is being taken in from the highway. It is impossible to completely eliminate the intake of outside air, since all cars produced since 1980 are constructed to have continuous fresh-air intake.

Although automotive ozone units for cars are now available to help decrease chemical odors, you should only buy one on the advice of your physician. Many of the newer models come equipped with air filters.

It may not always be possible for you to do so, but try to avoid rush-hour traffic, heavily traveled highways, frequent stoplight intersections, or other areas that have heavy exhaust accumulation. Plan your routes to avoid refineries, farms where insecticides are used, and large industrial plants. Try to remain at least four car lengths behind cars, trucks, and buses on the highway, particularly when they leave blue-gray exhaust smoke.

Leave your pets at home. Have the interior of your car vacuumed often. Clean floor mats to remove dust, pollens, and molds, and expose the mats to air and sunlight frequently to help prevent mold formation.

If you can find a full-service gas station, allow the attendant to pump the gas while you remain inside the car with the windows closed.

Although it is virtually impossible to completely purify your surroundings everywhere you go, at home, at work, and at play, you can choose between being a victim and being in control. You can discover ways to control your food, water, travel, and surroundings. You can choose to give up and give in, or you can choose to discover what causes your reactions and avoid the incitants that cause them. Since you're problems didn't develop overnight, chances are you're not going to reverse the process overnight either. Healing takes intentional, consistent, dedicated attention over a long period of time. There is no magic pill, but healing can happen. You can remain a functioning member of society. Don't retreat from life. Go out and face it on your own terms!

16

Chemicals to Avoid

FOUR GENERAL CATEGORIES of substances can induce multiple chemical sensitivity and trigger its symptoms. They are indoor air pollutants, outdoor pollutants, drug and consumer products, and food and water contamination.

Indoor air pollutants can include vapors emanating from solvents, paint, varnishes, adhesives, pesticides, white-out for office use, cleaning solutions, rubber cement, printing presses, and photocopiers. They can also include tobacco smoke, utility gas, perfumes and colognes, petrochemical contaminants, pesticides, fungicides, and gasses released from building materials such as particle board, fiberglass and insulation products, formaldehyde-containing pressboard, carpets, and plywood and plywood products. Sometimes they can be overlooked because they occur in simple, everyday items like coins and rubber bands, houseplants, epoxy glues, paper products, and such household polishes as furniture polish and even shoe polish. They can be the result of an infestation of common insects or the result of cold and heat, natural gas heat, and stoves or biological agents such as mold, mildew, and bacteria.

Formaldehyde is found in dry-cleaned and permanent-pressed clothing. It is also found in pressed-wood products such as plywood and chipboard. It is found in home furnishings that make use of plywood and chipboard in their construction as well as in carpets and upholstery fabrics.

Indoor air pollutants can be the unwelcome results of emissions from office supplies and equipment. Laser printers and copiers emit numerous chemicals. Computer terminals, laser printers, and dry-process copiers emit ozone, and typewriter correction fluid and some felt-tip markers emit volatile organic chemicals.

We all seem to be more familiar and aware of outdoor pollutants, which include such items as pesticides, automobile and diesel exhausts, industrial air pollutants, chemical waste disposal sites, vapors from paint manufacturing and sulfur-processing, fumes from roof and road tar, pollens, molds, and fragrant flora such as evergreens, flowers, and bushes.

Drug and consumer products can include medications, aspirin, barbiturates, sulfonamides, nonactive ingredients in drugs, mineral oils, petroleum jelly, laxatives, adhesive tape, most cosmetics, scented soaps, shampoos, hand lotions, perfumes and colognes, deodorants, hair sprays, hair dyes, mouthwashes, nail polishes and polish removers, hair spray, mousse, gel, denture adhesives, bath salts and oils, personal hygiene products, synthetic textiles, permanent-press finishes, detergents and fabric softeners, electric blankets (plastic coatings on wires release gases when heated), mattresses treated with flame retardant, books, magazines, newsprint, polishes, cleaners, and bleaches.

Food and water contaminants can come from insecticides and fumigant residues, some chemical preservatives and protective waxes, sulfur treatment, chemical flavorings, colorings and sweetening agents in foods, and artificial ripening procedures. Plastic containers used to store food and line cans contain a phenolic resin. Chlorine is present in treated water, and absorption is possible by bathing in the water as well as by drinking it.

There are some specific chemicals you will want to avoid. Phenol is also called carbolic acid. In 1845, the English surgeon Joseph Lister first used a dilute solution of phenol to treat wounds and established its use as an antiseptic. There are many hidden uses of phenol. It my be found as a constituent of herbicides and pesticides. It is used in the manufacturing of picric acid explosives. It serves as a starting point for the production of epoxy and phenolic resins as well as aspirin and other drugs. Phenol is also used in the manufacturing of nylon, synthetic detergents, polyurethane, many kinds of perfume, dyes, and photographic solutions. Phenol is commonly found as a sterilizing agent and disinfectant in household cleaners and disinfectants.

Bakelite, which is used in such frequently used molded articles as telephone parts, thermal insulation, panels and laminated boards, children's toys, and refrigerator storage dishes, is formed by the reaction of phenol with formaldehyde.

Phenol is used as a preservative in certain medications and as a preservative in some forms of immunotherapy. Weak phenolic compounds can be found in coal tar products such as certain skin medications and creosote. More than that, phenol occurs naturally as the toxic agent in poison ivy and poison oak, and it may occur naturally in spring water. Phenol irritates mucous membranes and can provoke severe immune responses. Phenols are poisonous to varying degrees. When they are present in sufficiently high doses, they can cause multiple tissue and organ damage and failure resulting in collapse, coma, or even death.

Alcohol is a class name used for a group of chemicals that include more than simply the commonly considered ethyl or drinking alcohol. Alcohol can be made from grains, grapes, or sugars. Industrial alcohol is sometimes made synthetically. In the US, industrial alcohol is generally made from corn, molasses, and sugars. Methyl alcohol is also called methanol or wood alcohol. It is highly toxic and is sometimes used to denature ethyl rubbing alcohol.

Ethyl alcohol is familiar as the alcohol formed as wine or hard cider by the fermentation of any sweet fruit juice, sugar cane, various grains, and sorghum. Much of the industrial ethyl alcohol in use is derived from chemical synthesis involving ethylene. Industrial ethyl alcohol can also be made from molasses, potatoes, or corn. Ethyl alcohol can dissolve many substances including shellac and oil. It is not only used as rubbing alcohol for the body; it is also used in making ether and in sterilizing surgical instruments. It is used extensively in making lacquers. It may also be found as an ingredient in tinctures and in many toiletry and drug preparations, hair sprays, and extracts such as vanilla or almond extract and the cola syrup used in soft drinks.

Amyl alcohol is made from ethyl alcohol and is used primarily in making lacquers and as flavoring in some foods.

Isopropyl alcohol is synthesized from propylene and is used to manufacture acetone. It is also used as a substitute for ethyl alcohol in manufacturing cosmetics, skin lotions, and rubbing alcohol.

Glycerol is used for making sweeteners and food preservatives. It is also used in manufacturing such diverse items as cosmetics, perfumes, inks, certain glues, explosives, paper, and antifreeze.

Menthol is used in manufacturing perfumes, confections, and liquors. Because of its cooling effect on mucous membranes, it is used in medications for colds and nasal disorders as well.

Ethylene glycol is used in making antifreeze and in making polyester fibers and plastics.

Formaldehyde is from a class of organic chemicals called aldehydes. It is a derivative of methanol that is used in industrial chemicals. In its pure form, it is a colorless gas with a pungent odor. It is highly toxic, even in very low concentrations. It accounts for approximately 50 percent of the estimated total aldehydes found in polluted air. Formaldehyde can become a significant indoor air pollutant. Specific concentrations can provoke eye irritations and respiratory irritations.

Several billion pounds of formaldehyde are produced each year in the United States. Because of its high chemical reactivity and physical-chemical properties, it is most often found and combined with other chemicals in the synthesis and production of a wide variety of products. Unreacted formaldehyde is also sometimes present in these products. It is virtually unavoidable in our modern industrialized environment. Primary sources of outdoor air concentrations include automotive and jet exhaust, emissions from industrial processes, photochemical smog, and gases released from urea-formaldehyde products.

A significant use of formaldehyde is in textile manufacturing, particularly in manufacturing permanent-press fabrics and artificial silk. It is used in combination with other chemicals to make natural and synthetic fibers crease resistant, wrinkle resistant, crushproof, dye fast, flame resistant, shrinkproof, water resistant, water repellent, mothproof, and more elastic. It can be used in the synthesis of dyes and in various specialty chemicals used in the dye industry. It also improves the color stability of dyed fabrics.

It is used extensively in the building industry, where it reduces shrinkage in wood and is important to the artificial aging of wood and wood veneer products. It is found in wood products, wood paneling, wallboard, plywood, particle board, pressboard, glues and resins, wallpaper, linoleum tile, floor and ceiling tile, electrical wiring, plastics, draperies, carpets and many other household products. It is used to make concrete, plaster and other products impermeable to liquids. The most common source of formaldehyde in the home is polyurethane foam insulation and carpet glues.

It is also used in the synthesis of alcohols, acids, and other chemicals and is employed to preserve such products as waxes, polishes, adhesives, fats, and oils. Its derivatives are also used in antiperspirants and as an antiseptic in dentifrices, mouthwashes, and germicidal and detergent soaps. It is used in hair styling products and shampoos and as resin in nail polish. Leather tanning agents also employ formaldehyde. It is important to the synthesis of vitamin A and for improving the activity of vitamin E preparations.

Formaldehyde is used in the formulation of slow-release nitrogen fertilizers and in destroying micro-organisms responsible for plant diseases. It can be used to destroy bacteria, fungi, molds, and yeast. It is used in insecticidal solutions for killing flies, mosquitoes, and moths and as a rodent poison.

It disinfects sickrooms and surgical instruments. It is also used in combination with alcohol, glycerol, and phenol in embalming fluids and is used to preserve anatomical specimens.

Exposure to formaldehyde comes primarily from inhaling and topical contact. It causes such health problems as upper respiratory tract irritation and burning, nose bleeds, and sore throats. It can cause lower respiratory tract irritation resulting in shortness of breath, chest tightness, in addition to wheezing, coughs, and asthma. It can also cause eye irritation, burning and excessive tears as well as skin irritations, burning, and rashes. Some responses to formaldehyde include headaches, dizziness, disorientation, mild memory loss and mood disorders, gastrointestinal distress, nausea, and vomiting. Severe allergic reactions can occur.

Pesticides are another common culprit in multiple chemical sensitivity. They are sprayed on farms, fields, lakes, forests, parks, lawns, and gardens. They are used in industrial and agricultural situations and extensively inside homes, schools, and workplaces. As a result of their widespread use, we have experienced damage to the food chain; reduced soil, water, and air quality; and the disruption of the stability and resilience of the world's ecosystem.

Pesticides can poison human cell metabolism and are toxic to the nervous system and immune system. Many people are highly allergic to pesticides. When they are exposed they risk immune reactions that can range from runny eyes and itching skin to muscle and joint pain to shock and even to death.

Many of the pesticides in common use today are chemically similar to the nerve gases developed during World War II and may be linked to the Desert Storm Syndrome.

Organochlorine (halogenated) compounds include such chemicals as polychlorinated biphenyls, carbon tetrachloride, freons, chloroethenes, chloroethanes, chloroethylenes, chlorobenzenes, dioxin, and such pesticides as DDT, chlordane, heptachlor, aldrin, dieldrin, and others. They have the ability to accumulate in animal and human fat tissue. Because of wide-scale pollution of our soil and water systems, they have found their way into our underground aquifers, streams, ponds, lakes, rivers and oceans, so that these compounds can be discovered almost everywhere. They occur in dairy products, meat, fowl, fish, produce, and in drinking water; they have even been found in human breast milk. They not only include halogenated pesticides but also certain industrial solvents and degreasers, herbicides, cleaning agents, dry cleaners and paint removers.

Many of these compounds have been confirmed as neurotoxic, hepatotoxic, cardiotoxic, nephrotoxic, and carcinogenic as a result of animal studies and incidents of acute human poisoning.

Petroleum products represent a major portion of a large class of chemicals called hydrocarbons. They comprise many toxic compounds including gasoline, kerosene, naphtha, benzene and benzene compounds, styrene, xylene, and toluene. They are used commonly as solvents, thinners, and cleansers and in the manufacture of rubber, resins, polyesters, and plastics. Also included are the by-products of incomplete organic combustion from petroleum, coal, and food. A major, although often unrecognized, source of petroleum byproducts is the result of outdoor cooking and barbecuing.

These products enter the environment through industrial waste, evaporation of solvents, and the burning of organic compounds, specifically as gasoline and diesel exhausts. They are also found occurring naturally as a result of the smoke from wood fires. Chronic exposure can result in vertigo; fatigue; nervousness; memory loss; nerve conduction abnormalities; chromosomal aberrations; severe bone marrow depression; leukemia; tissue death; fatty degeneration of the liver, heart, and adrenal glands; disease and degeneration of the brain; emotional problems; and certain cancers. There is also some evidence that toluene as well as other organic solvents may result in panic attacks in some people. Exposure to these chemicals usually occurs through inhalation, topical contact, and drinking water contamination.

Salicylates can be found in numerous prescription and nonprescription medications because they are effective anti-inflammatory agents, pain relievers, fever-lowering agents, and blood thinners. They include salicin, salicylic acid, methylsalicylate, and acetylsalicylic acid (better known as aspirin). Salicin occurs naturally in willow and poplar bark and oil of wintergreen.

Although aspirin is possibly the most often purchased and widely used over-the-counter drug in the United States, aspirin as well as all the salicylates can cause gastric irritation and upper gastrointestinal bleeding. It can also increase intestinal permeability to large protein molecules, promoting a more permeable, or "leaky," gut resulting in increased risk of developing further food hypersensitivities. Even when it is taken at normal daily doses, aspirin can cause tinnitis, decreased hearing, vertigo, and mild asymptomatic hepatitis.

The chemically sensitive person will have to make educated choices in avoiding toxic products. By making informed choices and by making environmental changes to accommodate specific sensitivities, you can live a more comfortable life.

Resources

By the time you reach this section of the book, you will have become aware of the choices and changes that can help you overcome the limits of your chemical sensitivity. Personal lifestyle changes can be most successful when you substitute less-toxic products for those that cause you to have reactions. After you have decided to make these lifestyles changes, it will become necessary for you to find sources for the products you want. While many of the less toxic products may be easily available in the general shopping locations in your area, some of the more specialized supplies may be difficult to locate.

This chapter of sources and resources is not meant to be a fully comprehensive source guide. You may not find some excellent sources that are specific to your locality, while others will be listed under several headings for your convenience. When possible, toll-free telephone numbers have been included. This source guide is designed to help you locate many of the things you will need so that you can substitute, not subsist, so that you can survive and thrive.

PRODUCTS TO HELP CLEAN THE AIR AROUND YOU

A+ Allergy Supply
8325 Regis Way
Los Angeles, CA 90045
(800) 86-ALLER

Aireox
1105 Whitford Ave.
Riverside, CA 92505
(797) 823-6202

Airguard Industries
PO Box 32578
Louisville, KY 40232
(502) 969-2304

Air Tech Equipment
(506) 532-0084

Allergy Alternative
440 Godfrey Dr.
Windsor, CA 95492-8036
(800) 838-1514

Allergy-Asthma Shopper
(800) 447-1100

The Allergy Store
PO Box 2555
Sebastopol, CA 95473
(707) 832-6202

AllerMed
31 Steel Rd.
Wylie, TX 75098
(214) 442-4898

Austin Air System
701 Seneca St.
Buffalo, NY 14210
(800) 724-8403
(716) 867-3704

Befit Enterprises Ltd.
PO Box 5034
Southampton, NY 11969
(800) 487-9516
(516) 287-3813

Berner Air Products
PO Box 5410-D
New Castle, PA 16105
(800) 852-5015

Bio-Tech Systems
4151 N. Kedzie
Chicago, IL 60618
(800) 612-5545

Bionaire Corporation
90 Boroline Rd.
Allendale, NJ 07401
(800) 253-2381

Clear Light
Box 551, State Rd. 165
Placitas, NM 87043
(505) 867-2381

Columbus Industries
2938 State Rte. 752
Ashville, OH 43103
(614) 983-2552

CYA Products, Inc.
211 Robins Ln.
Syosset, NY 11791
(516) 681-9394
FAX (516) 681-9395

D&J Trading Ltd.
PO Box 744
Lake Zurich, IL 60047
(708) 381-7058

Daliya Consulting Service
The Nontoxic Hotline
830 Meadow Rd.
Aptos, CA 95003
(800) You-Well
(408) 684-0199

The Dasun Co.
PO Box 668
Escondido, CA 92033
(800) 433-8929

Dust Free, Inc.
PO Box 519
Royce City, TX 75189
(214) 635-9565

E Group
PO Box 69
Fate, TX 75132
(800) 447-1167

Eco Source
PO Box 1656
Sebastopol, CA 95473
(800) 274-7040

EDI
4850 Northpark Dr.
Colorado Springs, CO 80918
(719) 599-9080

E.L. Foust Co., Inc.
Box 105
Elmhurst, IL 60126
(312) 834-4952

Enviracare
747 Bowman Ave.
Hagerstown, MD 21740 -6871
(800) 332-1110

Environment Now
PO Box 248
Yellow Springs, OH 45387

Environmental Air Purification
Systems
(817) 776-4878

Euroclean
907 W. Irving Park
Itasca, IL 60143
(800) 545-4372

Farr Company
2221 Park Place
El Segundo, CA 90245
(800) 4-FARRCO
(213) 772-5221

Flowright International Products
1495 NW, Gilman Blvd. #4
Issaquah, WA 98027
(106) 392-8357

For Your Health
6623 Hillandale Rd.
Chevy Chase, MD 20815
(301) 654-1127

Friederich Air Conditioning Co.
(800) 541-6645

Geothermal Energy Co.
PO Box 59
Wolfeboro, NH 25071
(304) 965-0482

Hi-Tech Filter Corp.
80 Myrtle St.
North Quincy, MA 02171
(617) 328-7758

Hurst
19C Monticello
Whiting, NJ 08759

Interior Air Quality
PO Box 3175
Grand Junction, CO 81502
(303) 242-3238

IOntertherm
(314) 822-9600

Life Support Resources
PO Box 738
Elkview, WV 25071
(301) 965-0482

The Living Source
7005 Woodway Dr. #214
Waco, TX 76712
(817) 776-4878

Lord & Kings, Inc.
PO Box 5496
Anderson, SC 29623
(803) 225-4782

Magr Industries
PO Box 1681
Welm, WA 98597
(206) 458-7455

Mother Hart's
PO Box 4229
Boynton Beach, FL 33427
(407) 738-5866
(407) 734-5942

Mountain Fresh Air
1560-1 Newbury Rd. #251
Newbury Park, CA 91320
(805) 498-6167

National Allergy Supply
(800) 522-1449

N.E.E.D.S.
527 Charles Ave.
Syracuse, NY 13209
(800) 534-1380
(315) 488-6300

New Dimensional Health
909 Montana
Belgrade, MT 59714
(406) 388-2473
(800) 598-5282

Newton Products Co.
3874 Virginia Ave.
Cincinnati, OH 45277
(800) 543-9149
(513) 561-7373

Nigra Enterprises
5699 Kanan Rd. 8CP
Agoura, CA 91303
(818) 889-6877

Nontoxic Environments
9392 S. Gribble Rd.
Canby, OR 97103
(503) 266-5244
FAX (503) 266-5242

Pac Chem Industries
779 S. La Grange Ave.
Newbury Park, CA 91320
(805) 499-1911

Packard Filter Co.
PO Box 178
Du Pont, WA 98327

Priorities
70 Walnut St.
Wellesley, MA 02181
(800) 553-5398

Pure Air Systems
Box 418
Plainfield, IN 46168
(800) 869-8025
FAX (317) 839-8567

Puridyne
2124 E. Hanna Ave.
Indianapolis, IN 46227
(800) 739-2444

Raschke, Christine
Sun River, MT 59483
(406) 264-5141

Real Goods
Ukiah, CA 95482-5507
(800) 762-7325
FAX (707) 468-9214

Safe House
724 Welch #11
Denton, TX 76201
(817) 382-3103

Safer Alternatives
19674 Day Lane
Redding, CA 96003
(916) 243-1352
FAX (916) 365-0601

Self Care Catalog
PO Box 182290
Chattanooga, TN 37422-7290
(800) 345-3371

Snyder General Corporation
215 Central Ave.
Louisville, KY 40232
(502) 637-0348

Thurmond Air Quality Systems
(800) AIR-PURE

Vent Air Systems
Colorado Springs, CO
(800) 777-VENT
(heat recovery ventilation systems)

Vitaire Corporation
PO Box 88
Elmhurst Annex, NY 11372 -0088

ALUMINUM FOIL

E.L. Foust Co. Inc.
PO Box 105
Elmhurst, IL 60126
(312) 834-4952

Living Source
7005 Woodway Dr. #214
Waco, TX 76712
(817) 776-4878

NonToxic Environments
9392 S. Gribble Rd.
Canby, OR 97103
(503) 266-5244
FAX (503) 266-5242

AUTOMOBILE PRODUCTS

Daliya Consulting Service
The Nontoxic Hotline
830 Meadow Rd.
Aptos, CA 95003
(800) YOU-WELL
(408) 684-0199

Magr Industries
PO Box 1681
Welm, WA 98597
(206) 458-7455

Packard Filter Co.
PO Box 178
Du Pont, WA 98327

Safe House
724 Welch #11
Denton, TX 76201
(817) 382-3103

Seventh Generation
Colchester, VT 05446-1672
(800) 456-1177
FAX (800) 456-1139

Zymol Enterprises
501 W. Pond Rd.
North Branford, CT 06471
(800) 999-5563

BEDS, BEDDING, AND PILLOWS

The Allergy Store
PO Box 2555
Sebastopol, CA 95473
(707) 832-6202

American Environmental Health
Foundation, Inc.
8345 Walnut Hill Lane #200
Dallas, TX 75231
(214) 361-9515

American Futons
PO Box 5396
Bloomington, IN 47057
(800) 821-8113

Bright Future
3120 Central Ave. SE
Albuquerque, NM
(505) 268-9738

The Company Store
500 Company Store Rd.
La Crosse, WI 54601
(800) 323-8000

The Cotton Place
PO Box 59721
Dallas, TX 75229
(800) 451-8866

Crown City Mattress
250 S. San Gabriel Blvd.
San Gabriel, CA 91776
(213) 681-6356
(818) 796-9101

Cuddledown of Maine
(800) 323-6793
FAX (207) 761-1948
E-mail: letter@cuddledown.com

Custom Bedding, Inc.
1677 Springfield Ave.
Maplewood, NJ 07040
(201) 674-1300

Dona Designs
835 Northlake Dr.
Richardson, TX 75080
(800) 235-0485

The Ecology Box
2260 S. Main St.
Ann Arbor, MI 48103
(800) 735-1371
(313) 662-9131

Eco Source
PO Box 1656
Sebastopol, CA 95473
(800) 274-7040

Garnet Hill
262 Main St.
Franconia, NH 03580
(800) 622-6216

Resources

Heart of Vermont
The Old Schoolhouse
Rte. 132, PO Box 183
Sharon, VT 05063
(800) 639-4123

Janice Corporation
198 Route 46
Budd Lake, NJ 07828
(800) 526-4237

Jantz Design
PO Box 371
Santa Rosa, CA 95402
(707) 823-8834

Karen's Nontoxic Products
1839 Dr. Jack Rd.
Conowingo, MD 21918
(800) 527-3674

KB Cotton Pillows
PO Box 57
De Soto, TX 75123
(800) 544-3752
(214) 223 -7193

The Living Source
7005 Woodway Dr. #214
Waco, TX 76712
(817) 776-4878

Mother Hart's
PO Box 4229
Boynton Beach, FL 33424
(407) 738-5866
(407) 734-5942

The Natural Bedroom
(800) 365-6563

NonToxic Environments
9392 S. Gribble Rd.
Canby, OR 97103
(503) 266-5244
FAX (503) 266-5242

Otis Bed Mfg.
Southgate Plaza
Union Rd.
W. Seneca, NY 14224
(716) 675-0238
or
University Plaza
3586 Main St.
Amherst, NY 14226
(716) 833-6712

Ozone
2340 E. 177th St.
Lansing, IL 60438
(708) 474-6166

Quilts, Etc.
938 Becky Circle
Hudson, WI 54016

Real Goods
(800) 762-7325
FAX (707) 468-9214

Safer Alternatives
19674 Day Ln.
Redding, CA 96003
(916) 243-1352
FAX (916) 365-0611

Seventh Generation
(800) 456-1777

Superior Mattress
(817) 834-2866

Vermont Country Store
PO Box 3000
Manchester Center, VT 05255-3000
(802) 362-2400

Wellness, Health & Pharmaceuticals
2800 S. 18th St.
Birmingham, AL 35209
(800) 227-2627

BOOKS

Bio-Probe
PO Box 608010
Orlando, FL 32860-8010
(800) 282-9670

Support Systems
Dept. OTT
Paron, AR 72122

Terra Verde
120 Wooster St.
New York, NY 10012
(212) 925-4533

BUILDING MATERIALS

Adams, Colway & Associates
412 Linden Ave.
Rochester, NY 14626
(800) 35-NYSEG
(Geothermal Heating)

AEHF
(800) 428-2343
(214) 361-9515

AFM Enterprises, Inc.
1140 Stacy Court
Riverside, CA 92507
(714) 781-6860

Air-Krete
Box 380
Weedsport, NY 13166
(315) 834-6609
(Insulation)

All Safe
5364 Pan American NE
Albuquerque, NM 87109
(Paint)

The Allergy Store
PO Box 2555
Sebastopol, CA 95473
(707) 832-6202

American Porcelain
(214) 637-4775
(Porcelain panels)

Anchor Paint
(214) 600-0151

Auro Paint-Sinan Co.
PO Box 857
Davis, CA 95617-0857
(916) 753-3104

Baubilogie Hardware
207 B 16th St.
Pacific Grove, CA 93950
(408) 372-8626

Bear Creek Lumber
PO Box 669
Winthrop, WA 98862
(509) 997-3110

Resources

Biofa Paints
PO Box 190
Alton, NH 03809

Bloom's Nontoxic Products
2442 Cerillos Rd. #207
Santa Fe, NM 87051
(505) 986-9222
Bonakemi, USA Inc.
14805 E. Moncrieff Pl.
Aurora, CO 80011
(800) 873-5515
(hardwood floor products)

Clear Life
PO Box 944
Mt. Shasta, CA 96067
(916) 926-2560

Design Materials, Inc
241 S. 55th St.
Kansas City, KS 66106
(800) 654-6451

Duo-Test Corp.
9 Law Dr.
Fairfield, NJ 07007
(800) 389-1515

Eco Paint
PO Box 375
St. Johnsbury, VT 05819
(802) 748-9144

EcoShop, Inc.
5884 E. 82nd St.
Indianapolis, IN 46250
(317) 84-WORLD

Eco Source
PO Box 1656
Sebastopol, CA 95473
(800) 274-7040

The Ecology Box
2260 S. Main St.
Ann Arbor, MI 48103
(800) 735-1371
(313) 662-9131

Enviro Clean
30 Walnut Ave.
Floral Park, NY
(800) 466-1425
(paint)

Environmental Construction Outfitter
44 Crosby St.
New York, NY 10012
(800) 238-5008
(212) 226-8084

Flowright International Products
1495 NW Gilman Blvd. #4
Issaquah, WA 98027
(206) 392-8357

Geothermal Energy Co.
PO Box 59
Wolfeboro, NH 25071
(304) 965-0482
(heat recovery)

Heavenly Heat
272 Neptune Ave.
Encinitas, CA 92024
(800) 533-0523
(Saunas)

Hendrickshon Naturlich
PO Box 1677
Sebastopol, CA 95473
(707) 824-0914
(flooring)

Henry Flack International
18333 Preston Rd., Ste. 460
Dallas, TX 75252
(800) 537-4929
(wood finishes)

Homasote
Box 7240
West Trenton, NJ 08626-0120
(800) 257-9491
(609) 883-3300
(paneling)

Karen's Nontoxic Products
1839 Dr. Jack Rd.
Conowingo, MD 21918
(800) 527-3674

The Living Source
7005 Woodway Dr. #214
Waco, TX 76712
(817) 776-4878

Major Paint Co.
4300 W. 190th St.
Torrance, CA 90509
(310) 542-7701

Mapes Industries
(800) 228-2391
(porcelain-on-aluminum panels)

Meadowood Industries
33242 Red Bridge Rd.
Albany, OR 97321
(503) 259-1303
(fiberboard)

Medite Corp.
PO Box 4040
Medford, OR 97501
(503) 773-2522
FAX (503) 779-9921
(fiberboard)

The Merchandise Mart
Merchandise Mart #1375
Chicago, IL 60654
(312) KITCHEN
(kitchens & baths)

Miller Paint Co.
317 SE Grand Ave.
Portland, OR 87214

Murco Wall Products
300 NE 21 St.
Fort Worth, TX 76106
(817) 626-1987

Nairn Floors International
560 Weber St. North
Waterloo, Ontario N2L 5C6
Canada
(519) 884-2602

Nontoxic Environments
9392 S. Gribble Rd.
Canby, OR 97103
(503) 266-5244
FAX (503) 266-5242

Nigra Enterprises
5699 Kanan Rd., SCP
Agoura, CA 91301
(818) 889-6877

Old Fashion Milk Paints Co.
PO Box 222
Groton, MA 10450
(508) 448-6336

Ozone
2340 E. 177th St.
Lansing, IL 60438
(708) 474-6166
(paints)

Pace Chem Industries
779 S. LaGrange Ave.
Newbury Park, CA 98136
(805) 449-2911

Palmer Industries, Inc.
10611 Annapolis Rd.
Frederick, MD 21701
(301) 898-7848
(insulation, paints, etc.)

Rainforest Harvest Eco-Wood
Finishes
Cultural Survival
11 Divinity St.
Cambridge, MA 02138
(617) 496-2562

RBM Logging & Lumber
PO Box 1105
Columbia Falls, MT 59912
(406) 892-4208

Safe House
724 Welch #11
Denton, TX 76201
(817) 382-3103

Safer Alternatives
19674 Day Lane
Redding, CA 96003
(916) 243-1352
FAX (916) 365-0611

Seventh Generation
Colchester, VT 05446-1672
(800) 877-2100

Solar Works
64 Main St.
Montpelier, VT 05602
(802) 223-7804

Thurmond Air Quality Systems
2512 Summit Ave.
Plano, TX 75074
(800) AIR-PURE
(214) 422-4000
Valhalla International Paints
RR1 Box 945
Craftsbury Commons, VT 05827

Valspar Corporation
200 Sayre St.
Rockford, IL 61101
(815) 987-3775

Vent-Aire Systems
4850 Northpark Dr.
Colorado Springs, CO 80918-3872
(800) 777-VENT
(719) 599-9080
(heat recovery ventilation systems)

W.R. Taylor Co., Inc
11545 Pacific Ave.
Fontana, CA 92335-8228
(adhesives)

Wood Finishing Supply
5604 Alameda Pine
Albuquerque, NM 87113 -2152

CATALOGS AND
MAIL ORDER SOURCES

AdaptAbility – Products for
Quality Living
(800) 288-9941

AEHF
(800) 428-2343
(214) 635-9840

Allergy-Asthma Shopper
(800) 447-1100

Allergy Relief Shop
(615) 522-2795

Biosys
(800) 821-8448
(415) 856-9506

CFIDS Health Buyers Club
(800) 366-6056

Conney Safety Products
Safety Catalog
(800) 356-9100

Cotton Place
(214) 243-4149

Deva Lifeware
PO Box 65
Westhope, ND 58793-0266
(800) 222-8024
FAX (800) 251-1746

Dona's Designs
1611 Burnt Tree St.
Seagoville, TX 75159

Eco Design-The Natural Choice
(800) 621-2591

Gardens Alive!
Organic Gardening Products
Sunman, IN
(812) 623-4201
FAX (812) 537-5108

Garden-Ville
(512) 288-6113

Good Friends Catalog
1025 W. 8th St., Dept. P
Kansas City, MO 64101-1200

Janice Corp.
(800) JANICES

The Living Source
7005 Woodway Dr. #214
Waco, TX 76712
(817) 776-4878

Mountain House Calls
Health Care Items
Ft. Worth, TX
(800) 460-7282

National Allergy Supply
(800) 522-1488
(404) 623-8077

The Natural Bedroom
(800) 365-6563

The Natural Choice
(505) 438-3448

Necessary Trading
(703) 864-5103

Nigra Enterprises
(818) 889-6877

Real Goods
(800) 762-7325

Seventh Generation
(800) 456-1177

Sinan Corp.
(916) 753-3104

Vermont Country Store
(802) 362-2400

Walnut Acres
Penn's Creek, PA 17862
(800) 433-3998

CHILD CARE PRODUCTS

The Allergy Store
PO Box 2555
Sebastopol, CA 95473
(707) 823-6202

The Company Store
500 Company Store Rd.
LaCrosse, WI 54601
(800) 323-8000

The Cotton Place
PO Box 59721
Dallas, TX 75229
(800) 451-8866

Garnet Hill
262 Main St.
Franconia, NH 03580
(800) 622-6216

Karen's Nontoxic Products
1839 Dr. Jack Rd.
Conowingo, MD 21918
(800) 527-3674

The Living Source
7005 Woodway Dr. #214
Waco, TX 76712
(817) 776-4878

Mother Hart's
PO Box 4229
Boynton Beach, FL 33424

(407) 738-5866
(407) 734-5924

Natural Baby Catalog
816 Silvia St.
Trenton, NJ 08628-3240
(800) 388-BABY

Seventh Generation
Colchester, VT
(800) 877-2100

Snugglebundle Enterprises
6325-9 Falls of Neuse Rd. #321
Raleigh, NC 27615

CLEANING AND
LAUNDRY PRODUCTS

The Allergy Store
PO Box 2555
Sebastopol, CA 95473
(707) 823-6202

American Environmental Health
Foundation
8345 Walnut Hill Lane, Ste. 200
Dallas, TX 75231
(214) 361-9515

Coastline Products
PO Box 6397
Santa Ana, CA 92706
(800) 554-4112
(800) 554-4111

Cultural Survival
11 Divinity St.
Cambridge, MA 02138
(617) 496-2562

Daliya Consulting Service
The Nontoxic Hotline
830 Meadow Rd.
Aptos, CA 95003
(800) YOU-WELL
(408) 684-0199

Dasun Company
PO Box 668
Escondido, CA 92033
(800) 433-8929

The Ecology Box
2260 S. Main St.
Ann Arbor, MI 48103
(800) 735-1371

Eco Shop Inc.
5884 E. 82nd St.
Indianapolis, IN 46250

Eco Source
PO Box 1656
Sebastopol, CA 95473
(800) 274-7040

Enviro-Clean
80 Walnut Ave.
Floral Park, NY 11001
(800) 466-1425

Heart of Vermont
The Old Schoolhouse
Rte. 132, PO Box 183
Sharon, VT 05063
(800) 639-4123

Karen's Nontoxic Products
1839 Dr. Jack Rd.
Conowingo, MD 20908
(800) 527-3674

The Living Source
7005 Woodway Dr. #214
Waco, TX 76712
(817) 776-4878

McDonnell & Co.
PO Box 815
East Granby, CT 06026
(800) 659-9177

Priorities
70 Walnut St.
Wellesley, MA 02181
(800) 553-5398

Schweitzer Enterprises
834 Spindle Hill Rd
Woolcott, CT 06716
(cleaning discs)

Seventh Generation
Colchester, VT 05446-1672
(800) 877-2100

Snowflake Laundry Soap
1725 Orrington Ave. #108-2
Evanston, IL 60201
(708) 332-9065

Walnut Acres
Penns Creek, PA
(800) 433-3998

Wellness, Health & Pharmaceuticals
2800 S. 18th St.
Birmingham, AL 35209
(800) 227-2627

Wendy's Naturals
603 Manor Ct.
Altoona, WI 54720
(715) 832-2992

Zymol Enterprises
50 W. Pond Rd.
N. Bramford, CT 06471
(800) 999-5563

CLOTHING AND LINGERIE

AEHF
(800) 428-2343
The Company Store
500 Company Store Rd.
LaCrosse, WI 54601
(800) 323-8000

The Cotton Place
PO Box 59721
Dallas, TX 75229
(800) 451-8866
(214) 243-4149

Cotton Threads Clothing
Rt. 2 Box 90
Hattlettsville, TX 77964
(409) 562-2153

Cottontails Organic Wear
3684 Hicks Hill Rd.
Friendship, NY 14739
(716) 973-3000

Deva Natural Clothes
Box 887
Burkittsville, MD 21718
(301) 663-4900

Dwina Originals
Salle A. Clark
1012 5th Ave. NW
Great Falls, MT 59404
(406) 452-5157

Eco Designs—The Natural Choice
(800) 621-2591

Ecosport
92 Kansas St.
Hackensack, NJ 07601
(800) 486-4326
(201) 489-0389

Eddie Bauer
(800) 426-8020

Garnet Hill
262 Main St.
Franconia, NH 03580
(800) 622-6216

Heart of Vermont
(800) 639-4123

J. Peterman Co.
2444 Palumbi Dr.
Lexington, KY 40509
(800) 231-7341

Janice Corporation
198 Rt. 46
Budd Lake, NJ 07828
(800) 526-4237

Land's End
1 Land's End Lane
Dodgeville, WI 53595
(800) 354-4444

Landau
114 Nassau St.
PO Box 671
Princeton, NJ 08542-0671
(800) 257-9445

The Living Source
7005 Woodway Dr. #214
Waco, TX 76712
(817) 776-4878

Ocarina Textiles
16-P Cliff St.
New London, CT 06320
(203) 437-8189

Organic Cotton
104 Clearfield Ln.
Coatsville, PA 19320
(215) 383-7774
FAX (215) 383-9951

Ozone
2340 E. 177th St.
Lansing, IL 60438
(708) 474-6166

Reflections Organic Clothing
Rt. 2, Box 24 P 40
Trinity, TX 75862
(409) 594-9019

Richman Cottons
(800) 992-8924

Seventh Generation
Colchester, VT 05446-1672
(800) 877-2100

Smith & Hawken
25 Corte Madera
Mill Valley, CA 94941
(415) 383-2000

Terra Verde
120 Wooster St.
New York, NY 10012
(212) 925-4533

Thai Silk
(800) 722-7455

Travis Place, Inc.
PO Box 30005
Durham, NC 27702-3005

(919) 682-3010
(800) 388-4101

Wearable Integrity
(310) 449-8606

Window Treatments & Women's
Clothing
402 N. 99th St.
Mesa, AZ 85207
(602) 373-9822

Winter Silks
2700 Laura Ln.
Middleton, WI 53562
(800) 648-7455

COMPUTER SCREENS AND COMPUTER PRODUCTS

Allergy-Asthma Shopper
(800) 447-1100

AEHF
(800) 428-2343

Allermed
(214) 442-4898

Baubiologie Hardware
(800) 447-1100

Real Goods
(800) 762-7325

Safe Computing Company
(800) 222-3003

FOOD

Sources for food that is organically grown in a chemical-free environment.

All of Washington's Best
16528 NE 35th Ct., Ste. QQ103
Redmond, WA 98052
(206) 869-2984

Bandon's Sea Pack
PO Box 5488
Charleston, OR 97420
(800) 255-4370
(503) 888-4600

Chuck's Seafood
(503) 888-4600

Clear Eye Natural Foods
302 Rt. 89 S.
Savannah, NY 13146
(800) 724-2233

Colorado Prime Meat
(303) 553-1411

Crosssroad Farm
Box 3230
Jonesport, ME 04649
(207) 487-2641

Czimer Foods
Rte #10, Box 285
Lockport, IL 06441
(312) 460-2210

DeBole's Natural Foods
2120 Jericho Turnpike
Garden City Park, NY 11040
(516) 742-1818

Eco Bella
The Environmental Store
(800) 888-5320

The Ecology Box
2260 S. Main St.
Ann Arbor, MI 48103

(800) 735-1371
(313) 662-9131

Ecology Sound Farms
42126 Road 168
Orosi, CA 93647
(209) 528-3816

Food Care
(217) 687-5115

French Meadow Bakery
2160 Lyndale Ave. S.
Minneapolis, MN 55408
(612) 870-4740

The Green Earth
2545 Prairie
Evanston, IL 60201
(800) 332-3662

Horak Farms, Inc.
1217 200th St.
Hubbard, NE 68741

Harbor House Organic Coffee
PO Box 1879
Clearlake Oaks, CA 95423
(800) 541-4699

H&M Natural Foods
(214) 231-6083

Hans Mueller
(214) 241-1107

Horseshoe Hollow Farm
Washington, VA 22747
(703) 675-3165

Jaffe Bros. Inc.
(619) 749-1133

Kennedy
(703) 533-8488

The Living Source
7005 Woodway Dr. #214
Waco, TX 76712
(800) 662-8787

The Meat Shop
13419 Vickery Ave. East
Tacoma, WA 98446
(206) 537-4490
Mountain Ark Trading Co.
PO Box 3170
Fayetteville, AR 72702-3170
(800) 643-8909
FAX (501) 521-9100

Mountain Valley Food
404 1st Ave. East
Kalispell, MT 59901
(406) 756-1422

Natural Beef Farm
(703) 631-0881

Olde World Coffee Co.
9514 SW 140th Ct.
Miami, FL 33186
(800) 846-6979

Organic Food Shopper
1578 W. Lewis, Dept. E.
San Diego, CA 92103
(619) 425-2813

Organic Wholesaler's Directory
& Yearbook
Box 464
Davis, CA 95617

Organic Wine Works
(800) 699-WINE
(408) 335-4441

Orange Blossom Co-op
1601 NW 55th Pl.
PO Box 4159
Gainesville, FL 32613
(904) 372-7061

Oshwa America Macrobiotic Foods
PO Box 3608
Chico, CA 95927
(916) 342-6050
Purity Foods
2871 W. Jolly Rd.
Okemos, MI 48864
(517) 351-9231

Rue, Betty L.
PO Box 66
Roundup, MT 59072

Special Foods
9207 Shotgun Ct.
Springfield, VA 22153
(703) 644-0991

Sunrise Health Food Store
17650 Torrence
Lansing, IL 60438
(708) 474-6166

Totality
(619) 425-2813

Traditional Provisions
412 N. Fairfax Blvd.
Ranson, WV 25438
(304) 725-6322

Under the Sun
PO Box 633
Winters, CA 95694
(916) 795-5256

Vermont Country Store
PO Box 3000
Manchester Center, VT 05255-3000
(802) 362-2400

Walnut Acres
Dept. 1120
Penn's Creek, PA 17862
(800) 433-3998

Weatherby Beef
(915) 372-3324

Wild Games, Inc.
2315 W. Huron
Chicago, IL 60612
(312) 278-1661

Whole Foods Market, Inc.
(512) 477-4455

FURNITURE

Clearlife Industries
PO Box 277
Mt. Shasta, CA 96067
(916) 926-2460
(canvas recliners)

Dona's Designs
825 Northlake Rd.
Richardson, TX 75080
(800) 235-0485
(pillows, chair covers)

Heart of Vermont
The Old Schoolhouse
Rte 132, Box 183
Sharon, VT 05065
(800) 630-4123

HEATING AIR CONDITIONING SYSTEMS

You will want to avoid gas floor or wall furnaces, unvented gas heaters, wood stoves, improperly vented fuel-fired furnaces, or any system that exposes users to natural gas or gas combustion by-products. These sources can provide a variety of systems. You may wish to install metal ductwork with vapor barrier and insulation on the outside, electric baseboard or forced-air heat with power sources in the attic or basement. You may wish to install a fuel-fired furnace that is located six feet away from the house or in a basement or sealed room and is vented to the outside. Heat pumps should be installed with motor outside the airstream.

Adams Colway & Associates
412 Linden Ave.
Rochester, NY 14626
(800) 35-NYSEG
(geothermal heating)

Ceramic Radiant Heat
PO Box 60
Greenport, NY 11944
(800) 331-6408

Daliya Consulting Service
The Nontoxic Hotline
830 Meadow Rd.
Aptos, CA 95003
(800) YOU-WELL
(408) 684-0199

Intertherm
(314) 822-9600

The Living Source
(800) 662-8787
(817) 776-4878

Nigra Enterprises
5699 Kanan Rd. 8 CP
Agoura, CA 91301
(818) 889-6877

Nontoxic Environments
9392 S. Gribble Rd.
Canby, OR 97103
(503) 266-5242
FAX (503) 266-5242

Radiant Heater Corp.
PO Box 60
Greenport, NY 11944
(800) 331-6408

Real Goods
(800) 762-7325
(solar systems)

Zell-Air
(215) 372-9579

HOUSEWARES

Curtains, shower curtains, cotton per-
cale sheets, cotton and wool blankets,
cotton and wool pillows, etc.

AEHF
(800) 428-2343
(214) 361-9515

Allergy-Asthma Shopper
(800) 447-1100
(214) 635-9840

Atlanta Recycled Paper
Box 39179
Baltimore, MD 21212
(800) 323-2811

Chambers
(800) 334-9790

The Cotton Place
PO Box 59721
Dallas, TX 75229
(800) 451-8866

Dona's Designs
1611 Bent Tree St.
Seagoville, TX 75159

Dwina Originals
Sally A. Clark
1012 5th Ave. NW
Great Falls, MT 59404
(406) 452-5157

Eddie Bauer
(800) 426-8020

Garnet Hill
262 Main St.
Franconia, NH 03580
(800) 622-6216

Heart of Vermont
(800) 639-4123
(802) 763-2720

Janice Corporation
198 Rte. 46
Budd Lake, NJ 07828
(800) 526-4273

Karen's Nontoxic Products
1839 Dr. Jack Rd.
Conowingo, MD 21918
(800) 527-3674

The Living Source
(800) 662-8787
(817) 776-4878

The Natural Bath
PO Box 97
Haddonfield, NJ 08033
(609) 427-1005

The Natural Bedroom
(800) 365-6563

Non Polluting Enterprises, Inc.
PO Box 919 DD
Old Chelsea Station
New York, NY 10011
(800) 782-NOPE

Nontoxic Environments
9392 S. Gribble Rd.
Canby, OR 97103
(503) 266-5244
FAX (503) 266-5242

Real Goods
(800) 762-7325

Terra Verde
120 Wooster St.
New York, NY 10012
(212) 925-4533

Vermont Country Store
PO Box 3000
Manchester Center, VT 05255-3000
(802) 362-4667

Window Treatments & Women's
Clothing
402 N. 99th St.
Mesa, AZ 85207
(602) 373-9823

LIGHT, FULL-SPECTRUM

Nontoxic Environments
9392 S. Gribble Rd.
Canby, OR 97103
(503) 266-5244

Park Industrial Lighting
375 7th Ave. NW
Kalispel, MT 59901
(406) 752-8396

Randal Electric Company
9215 1st St.
Berrien Springs, MI 49103
(616) 471-1534

Seventh Generation
Colchester, VT 05446-1672
(800) 877-2100

Vitality Concepts, Inc.
1406 W. Summerdale Ave.
Chicago, IL 60640-2116
(312) 275-1443

MAGAZINES

Delicate Balance
(609) 429-5358

Delicate Balance
(609) 429-5358

Human Ecologist
(404) 248-1898

Natural Food & Farming
NFA
PO Box 210
Atlanta, TX 75551
(800) 594-2136

Our Toxic Times
Chemical Information Network
PO Box 301
White Sulfer Springs, MT 59654

20th Century Living
PO Box 354
Forestburg, TX 76239

Karen's Nontoxic Products
(800) 527-3674

The Living Source
7005 Woodway Dr. #214
Waco, TX 76712
(817) 776-4878

Real Goods
(800) 762-7325

Wellness, Health & Pharmaceuticals
(800) 227-2627

MAKE-UP

Alexandra Avery
(503) 766-2446
(sunscreen with PABA and sesame oil)

The Allergy Store
PO Box 2555
Sebastopol, CA 95473
(707) 823-6202

The Cotton Place
(800) 451-8866

Eco Bella, The Environmental Store
(800) 888-5320

Eco Design –The Natural Choice
(800) 621-2591
(sunscreen for children)

Eco Source
(800) 274-7040

Granny's
(800) 428-2343
(214) 361-9515

MASKS

American Environmental Health
Foundation
8345 Walnut Hill Lane, Ste. 200
Dallas, TX 75231
(214) 361-9515

The Dasun Co.
PO Box 668
Escondido, CA 92033
(800) 433-8929

Denbraber, Sandy
114 Ray St.
Arlington, TX 70610
(817) 776-4878

E.P.S. Environmental Purification
Systems
(415) 284-2129
(ceramic masks)

The Living Source
7005 Woodway Dr. #214
Waco, TX 76712
(817) 776-4878

McMillian, Martha
905 E. Buffalo Ave. Dept. H.
Santa Ana, CA 92706
Nontoxic Environments
9392 S. Gribble Rd.
Canby, OR 97103
(503) 266-5242
FAX (503) 266-5242

Safer Alternativies
19674 Day Ln.
Redding, CA 96003
(916) 243-1352

ORGANIZATIONS

The American Academy of
Environmental Medicine
4510 West 89th St.
Prairie Village, KS 66207-2218
(903) 642-6062
(information about environmental
medicine. Also has lists of all the
doctors in the U.S. who practice
environmental medicine.)

The Environmental Health Center
(214) 373-5146
(environmental alternatives
consultation)

Environmental and Preventative
Health Center of Atlanta
Dr. Stephen Edelson, MD
3833 Roswell Rd., Ste. 110
Atlanta, GA 30342–4432
(404) 841-0088

The Environmental Protection
Agency (EPA)
(800) 438-4318

("Tools for Schools," is an action kit
with practical advice for healthy
schools.)

HEAL
(404) 248-1898

National Center for Environmental
Health Strategies
(609) 429-5358

National Institute of Environmental
Health Sciences
Environmental Health Clearinghouse
(800) 643-4794

NIOSH (National Institute of
Occupational Safety and Health
Information)
(800) 356-4674
(information hotline answers questions about health problems in the
workplace)

OXYGEN EQUIPMENT AND
SUPPLIES

American Environmental Health
Foundation
8345 Walnut Hill Ln., Ste. 200
Dallas, TX 75231
(214) 361-9515

E.P.S. (Environmental Purification
Systems)
(415) 284-2129

The Living Source
7005 Woodway Dr. #214
Waco, TX 76712
(817) 776-4878

PAPER AND PAPER PRODUCTS

AEHF
(800) 428-2343
(214) 361-9515
(nontoxic art supplies, crayons, chalk,
fingerpaints)

Atlanta Recycled Paper
PO Box 39179
Baltimore, MD 21212
(800) 323-2811
(410) 323-2676

Earth Care Paper
PO Box 7070
Madison, WI 53707
(608) 277-2900

Eco Bella
The Environmental Store
(800) 888-5320

Eco Designs – The Natural Choice
(800) 621-2591
(505) 438-3448
(nontoxic art supplies, crayons, chalk,
fingerpaints)

The Eco Shop
1884 E. 82nd St.
Indianapolis, IN 46250
(317) 84-WORLD

Lynn-Bar Enterprises & Graphic
Exposure Designs
33 Plandome Rd.
Manhassett, NY 11030
(516) 365-6961

Niagara of WI Paper Corp.
1101 Mill St.
Niagara, WI 54151
(800) 826-0432

Peterson's
Rte 1 Box 176
Oronogo, MO 64855
(thank-you cards)

Sagewood Stationary
1101 Crazy Woman Canyon Rd.
Buffalo, WY 82834
(800) 788-4672

Seventh Generation
Colchester, VT 05466-1672
(800) 877-2100

Terra Verde
120 Wooster St.
New York, NY 10012
(212) 935-4533

Treecycle Recycled Paper
PO Box 5086
Bozeman, MT 59715
(406) 586-5287

PERSONAL HYGIENE

Allergy Alternative
440 Godfrey Dr.
Windsor, CA 95492-8036
(800) 838-1514

The Allergy Store
PO Box 2555
Sebastopol, CA 95473
(707) 823-6202

American Environmental Health
Foundation
8345 Walnut Hill Lane, Ste. 200
Dallas, TX 75231
(214) 361-9515

Resources

Aubrey Organics
4419 N. Manhattan Ave.
Tampa, FL 33614
(800) 282-7394

Body Elements
3320 N. 3rd St.
Arlington, VA 22201-1712
(703) 525-0585

The Body Shop
45 Horsehill Rd.
Cedar Knolls, NJ 07927-2003
(800) 541-2535

Bull Mountain Made
809 Bench
Billings, MT 59105
(406) 252-9027

Caring for You
1139 Cotswald Ct.
Sunnyvale, CA 94087
(408) 296-7968

Coastline Products
PO Box 6397
Santa Ana, CA 92706
(800) 554-4111 (orders)
(800) 554-4112 (customer service)

The Cotton Place
(800) 451-8866

Eco Bella, The Environmental Store
(800) 888-5320

Eco Design – The Natural Choice
(800) 621-2591

The Ecology Box
2260 S. Main St.
Ann Arbor, MI 48103

(800) 735-1371
(313) 662-9131

Eco Shop, Inc.
5884 E. 82nd St.
Indianapolis, IN 46250
(317) 84-WORLD

Eco Source
(800) 274-7040

Flowright International Products
1495 NW Gilman Blvd. #4
Issaquah, WA 98027
(206) 392-8357

Granny's E2
3581 E. Milton St.
Pasadena, CA 91107
(800) 428-2343
(214) 361-9515

Home Health Products
1160 A Miller's Lane
Virginia Beach, VA 23451
(800) 284-9123

Janice Corporation
198 Rte. 46
Budd Lake, NJ 07828
(800) 526-4237

Karen's Nontoxic Products
Conowingo, MD
(800) 527-3674

The Living Source
7005 Woodway Dr. #214
Waco, TX 76712
(817) 776-4878

Logona USA
580-B Dutch Valley Rd.
Atlanta, GA 30324
(800) 648-6654

New Cycle Products, Inc.
PO Box 17875
Sebastopol, CA 95473
(707) 829-2744
FAX (707) 829-1753
(sanitary napkins)

Non Polluting Enterprises, Inc.
(800) 782-NOPE

Nontoxic Environments
9392 S. Gribble Rd.
Canby, OR 97103
(503) 266-5244
FAX (503) 266-5242

Real Goods
(800) 762-7325

Reviva Cosmetic Labs
(800) 257-7774

Seventh Generation
(800) 877-2100

Wellness, Health & Pharmaceuticals
(800) 227-2627

PESTICIDES, HERBICIDES, AND ALTERNATIVES

Arborist, Alternatives to Pesticides
Box 381
Elmbridge, NY 13060
(315) 689-3288

Avert
(812) 537-8650
(abamectin insecticidal bait)

Biofac, Inc.
PO Box 36
Mathis, TX 78368
(512) 547-3259
(fire ants)

Biological Control of Weeds
1140 Cherry Dr.
Bozeman, MT 59715
(406) 586-5111

Biosys
(800) 821-8448

Bora Care
(800) 264-0870
(termites)

Carpet Stuff
(800) 456-1177
(fleas and ticks in carpets and upholstery)

Earth Dynamics
(713) 575-0112

Eco-Science
(800) 998-2467
(fungal roach bait)

Eco Source
PO Box 16756
Sebastopol, CA 954473
(800) 274-7040

Environmental Health Center
(information on pesticides)
(214) 373-7139

Resources

Flea Busters
(800) 666-3532

Gardens Alive
(812) 537-8650
(garden and lawn pests)

Gardenville
(912) 537-8650
(garden and lawn pests)

Karen's Nontoxic Products
1839 Dr. Jack Rd.
Conowingo, MD 21918
(800) 527-3674

Lakon Herbals
RR1 Box 4710
Templeton Rd.
Montpelier, VT 05602

The Living Source
7005 Woodway Dr. #214
Waco, TX 76712
(817) 776-4878

Motherwater
PO Box 114
Northampton, MA 01061
(413) 586-3488

National Coalition Against Misuse
of Pesticide
(information on pesticides)
(202) 544-2600

Natrapel
(802) 863-1700
(mosquito repellant containing aloe
vera and citronella)

Natural Animal
(800) 274-7387

(herbal pet collar, pet shampoo, flea
products)

Natural Gardening Research Center
PO Box 149
Sunman, IN 47041
(812) 623-4201
(fire ant hormone bait)

Necessary Trading Co.
PO Box 305
New Castle, VA 24127
(800) 447-5354

Nitron Industries
(800) 835-0123

Organic Pest Control
PO Box 55223
Phoenix, AZ 85087

Peaceful Valley Farm Supply
(916) 272-4769

Perfectly Safe
(800) 837-KIDS

Pesticide Hotline
(information on pesticides)
(800) 858-7378

Prince Lionheart
2421 Whipple Ave. NW
Santa Maria, CA 93455
(800) 544-1132

Pristine Products
2311 E. Indian School Rd.
Phoenix, AZ 85016
(800) 266-4968
(602) 955-7031

Reemer Insecticidal Soap
(812) 537-8650
(512) 892-0704

Ringer Products
9959 Valley View Rd.
Eden Prairie, MN 55344
(612) 829-5430

Seventh Generation
(800) 428-0412

Simmons Handcrafts
42295 Hwy. 36
Bridgeville, CA 95621
(800) 428-0412
(916) 961-7945

Skeeter Off
(802) 623-3800
(natural mosquito repellant)

Unique Insect Control
5504 Sperry Dr. Dept. GA
Citrus Heights, CA 95621
(916) 967-7082
FAX (916) 967-7082

U.S.D.A. Forest Lab
(601) 864-3991
(information on pesticides; tests all
forms of termite treatment)

Walnut Acres
(800) 433-3998
(512) 892-0704

PET CARE PRODUCTS

A+ Allergy Supply
(800) 86-ALLER

All the Best
2714 E. Madison
Seattle, WA 98112
(800) 771-2246

American Environmental Health
Foundation
8345 Walnut Hill Lane, Ste. 200
Dallas, TX 75231
(214) 361-9515

Body Elements
3320 N. 3rd St.
Arlington, VA 22201-1712
(703) 525-0585

Pristine Products
(800) 266-4YOU

Seventh Generation
(800) 877-2100

Wendy's Naturals
603 Manor Ct.
Altoona, WI 54720
(715) 832-2992

READING AND COMPUTER BOXES

ALLERMED
31 Steel Rd.
Wylie, TX 75098
(214) 442-4898

AEHF
(800) 428-2343

Allergy-Asthma Shopper
(800) 447-1100

The Living Source
7005 Woodway Dr. #214
Waco, TX 76712
(817) 776-4878

Safe Reading & Computer Boxes Co.
(517) 687-3989

RUGS, CARPETING, AND FLOORING

Carousel Carpet Mills
(707) 485-0333

Chambers Co.
(800) 334-9790

Desso Carpet
(800) 368-1515

Gladys Rugs
1790 Wynkoop St.
Denver, CO 80202
(800) 658-8056

Heart of Vermont
(800) 639-4123

Janice Corporation
(800) 526-4237

Laura Copenhaver
(800) 227-6797

Monarch Trading Co.
(800) 367-6002

The Natural Bedroom
(800) 365-6563

Naturlich Flooring
(800) 329-9398

Nontoxic Environments
(503) 266-5224

Real Goods
(800) 762-7325

Seventh Generation
(800) 456-1177

SHOES, SLIPPERS, AND BOOTS

AEHF
(800) 428-2343

The Cotton Place
(800) 451-8866

J. Peterman, Co.
(800) 231-7341

Janice Corporation
(800) 526-4237

Heart of Vermont
(800) 630-4123

Ozone
2340 E. 177th St.
Lansing, IL 60438
(708) 474-6166

Richmond Cotton Co.
(800) 992-8924

Smith & Hawken
25 Corte Madera
Mill Valley, CA 94901
(415) 383-2000

Swedish Clogs, Inc.
(800) 443-8167

Vermont Country Store
PO Box 3000
Manchester Center, VT 05255-3000

SMOKE ALARMS

Allergy-Asthma Shopper
(800) 447-1100

Real Goods
(800) 762-7325

Eco Design – The Natural Choice
(800) 621-2591

TOYS AND BOOKS FOR CHILDREN

Art & Craft Material Institute
715 Boylston St.
Boston, MA 02116
(child-safe art supplies)

Crate & Barrel
PO Box 3057
Northbrook, IL 60065
(800) 323-5461
(wooden toys)

Eco Design – The Natural Choice
(800) 621-2591

Heart of Vermont
(800) 639-4123

Hearth Song
170 Professional Center Dr.
Rohnerst Park, CA 94928-2149

K&D Specialties
119 1/2 Cypress
Wallace, ID 83873

Karen's Nontoxic Products
1839 Dr. Jack Rd.
Conowingo, MD 21918
(800) 527-3674

Seventh Generation
(800) 877-2100

VACUUM CLEANERS

A+ Allergy Supply
8325 Regis Way
Los Angeles, CA 90041
(800) 86-ALLER

Daliya Consulting Service
The Nontoxic Hot Line
830 Meadow Rd.
Aptos, CA 95003
(800) YOU-WELL
(408) 684-0199

Hydro Life, Inc.
503 Maple St.
Bristol, IN 46507
(800) 626-7130

Mountain Air Hygenics
PO Box 225
Newton, MA
(800) 533-4028

Nigra Enterprises
5699 Kanan Rd. SCP
Agoura, CA 91301
(818) 889-6877

The Nontoxic Hotline
830 Meadow Rd.
Aptos, CA 95003
(800) YOU-WELL
(408) 684-0199

Priorities
70 Walnut St.
Wellesley, MA 02181
(800) 552-5398

VITAMINS, MINERALS, AND HOLISTIC MEDICATIONS

Allergy Alternative
440 Godfrey Dr.
Windsor, CA 95492-8036
(800) 838-1514

Allergy Research Group
400 Pedra St.
San Leandro, CA 84577
(800) 545-9960

The Allergy Store
PO Box 2555
Sebastopol, CA 95473
(707) 832-6202

American Environmental Health
Foundation
8345 Walnut Hill Lane, Ste. 200
Dallas, TX 7531
(214) 361-9515

Bio-Probe
PO Box 608010
Orlando, FL 32860-8010
(800) 282-9670

Body Wise
Beth McCluskie
3325 Saunders Rd. #26
Laramie, WY 82070
(307) 742-7968

Caring for You
1139 Cotswald Ct.
Sunnyvale, CA 94087
(408) 296-7968

Eco Source
PO Box 1656
Sebastopol, CA 95473
(800) 274-7040

Engen Drug Allergy Div.
PO Box 218
Karlstad, MN 56732
(800) 658-0074
(218) 436-2485

Health Comm.
5800 Soundview Dr.
PO Box 1729
Gig Harbor, WA 98355
(800) 648-5883

Home Health Products
1160 A Millers Lane
Virginia Beach, VA 23451
(800) 284-9123

Karen's Nontoxic Products
1839 Dr. Jack Rd.
Conowingo, MD 21918
(800) 527-3674

L & H Vitamins
37-10 Crescent Ct.
Long Island City, NY 11001
(800) 221-1152

The Living Source
7005 Woodway Dr. #214
Waco, TX 76712
(817) 776-4878

Mountain Pure Products
(800) 359-9575

Mountain Rose Herbs
PO Box 2000
Redway, CA 95560
(800) 522-8929

Nature's Balance
10705 N. Main St.
Archdale, NC 27263
(800) 858-5198

N.E.E.D.S.
527 Charles Ave.
Syracuse, NY 13209
(800) 534-1380
(315) 488-6300

Neo-Life Alternative
207 North Shore Dr.
Cary, IL 60013

Nontoxic Environments
9392 S. Gribble Rd.
Canby, OR 97103
(503) 266-5244
FAX (503) 266-5242

Specialty Organic Source
PO Box 1628
Champaign, IL 61824
(800) 782-5581

Sunrise Health Food Store
17650 Torrence
Lansing, IL 60438
(708) 474-6166

Swan Valley Natural Health and
Herbal Pharmacy
PO Box 282
Bigfork, MT 59911
(406) 837-5747

Wellness, Health & Pharmaceuticals
2800 S. 18th St.
Birmingham, AL 35209

WATER

County Health Department
Your county health department can
analyze the drinking water in your
home to tell you which specific contaminants are present.

Environmental Health Clearinghouse
(800) 643-4794
Information on health effects of particular contaminants, on home water
treatment units and prices, and on
locating a certified drinking water laboratory in your area.

National Sanitation Foundation
(313) 769-8010
An independent testing laboratory
that certifies particular products for
specific uses.

Water Quality Association
(312) 369-1600
To ensure that you are getting satisfactory quality and a desirable level of
effectiveness in your home water
treatment system, you might look for
the insignia of the Water Quality
Association on your product. This
trade association is made up of distrib-
utors and manufacturers. It offers its
members voluntary validation standards and advertising guidelines.

Water distillers

Eco Water Systems
PO Box 64420
St. Paul, MN 55164

Purity Products
PO Box 437
Depew, NY 14043
(716) 683-7079

Rain Crystal Products
113 Phoenix Ave. NW
Albuquerque, NM 87125
(505) 345-7321

Resources

Safer Alternatives
19674 Day Lane
Redding, CA 96003
(916) 243-1325
FAX (916) 365-0611

Scientific Glass
113 Phoenix NW
Albuquerque, NM 87107
(404) 874-8700

Waterwise, Inc
26200 U.S. Hwy. 27
Leesburg, FL 34748
(800) 874-9028
(904) 787-5008

Water purifiers

A+ Allergy Supply
8325 Regis Way
Los Angeles, CA
(800) 86-ALLER

AEHF (Aqua Clear)
(800) 428-2343

Allergy Alternative
440 Godfrey Dr.
Windsor, CA 95492-8036
(800) 838-1514

Allergy-Asthma Shopper
(800) 447-1100

The Allergy Store
PO Box 2555
Sebastopol, CA 95473
(707) 823-6202

Bio-Tech Systems
4151 N. Kedzie
Chicago, IL 60618
(800) 612-5545

Calgon Carbon Corporation
PO Box 717
Pittsburgh, PA 15230-0717
(800) 422-7266

Clean-Flo Laboratories, Inc.
4342 Shady Oak Rd.
Hopkins, MN 55343
(612) 935-2138

Cuno
400 Research Parkway
Meriden, CT 06540
(203) 237-5541

Daliya Consulting Service
The Nontoxic Hotline
830 Meadow Rd.
Aptos, CA 95003
(800) YOU-WELL
(408) 684-0199

Eco Source
PO Box 1656
Sebastopol, CA 95473
(800) 274-7040

Everpure
(312) 654-4000

Flowright International Products
1495 NW Gilman Blvd. #4
Issaquah, WA 98027
(206) 392-8357

Fluid Mechanics Inc.
2781 Klondike Rd.
W. Lafayette, IN 47906-5220

Global Environmental Technologies
Box 8839
Allentown, PA 18105
(800) 284-9123

Home Health Products
1160 A Millers Lane
Virginia Beach, VA 23451
(800) 284-9123

Hydro Life, Inc.
503 Maple St.
Bristol, IN 46507
(800) 626-7130

The Living Source
7005 Woodway Dr. #214
Waco, TX 76712
(817) 776-4878

N.E.E.D.S.
527 Charles Ave.
Syracuse, NY 13209
(800) 634-1380
(315) 488-6320

Ozark Analytical Water Lab
114 Springs St.
Sulpher Springs, AR 72768
(800) 835-8908
(501) 298-3483

Pacific Environmental
931 Metro Dr.
Monterey Park, CA 91754
(800) 243-8775

Personal Dimensions
PO Box 1381
Healdsburg, CA 95448
(707) 433-8774

Pura-Tech
PO Box 298
Groveport, OH 43125
(614) 836-9422

The Pure Water Place
PO Box 6715

Longmont, CO 80501
(303) 776-0056

Pure Water West
272 Srowl Creek Rd.
Garberville, CA 95440
(800) 824-1555

R.H. of Texas
PO Box 780392
Dallas, TX 75378
(214) 368-4132

Safe House
724 Welch #11
Denton, TX 76201
(817) 382-3103

Scale Watcher Inc.
(215) 384-7200

Scientific Glass
(505) 345-7321

Waterwise, Inc
Leesburg, FL
(800) 874-9028

Portable water purifiers

Purifying Water Straw
(800) 878-2580

Recovery Engineering
2229 Edgewood Ave. South
Minneapolis, MN 55425-2822
(800) 845-PURE

Water Technologies Corporation
14405 21st Ave. North
Plymouth, MN 55447
(612) 473-1625

Index

Index

Index

need for reasonable accommodations in, 84–85

often asked questions about, 1–3

and pollution, 21–27

risks for, 41–43

role of government in dealing with, 102–5

setting up personal oasis in, 163–67

spread of, 2, 16–17

switching in, 17–18

symptoms of, 3, 27, 67–69, 81–82, 149

timing of, 2–3

total body load in, 10–11

treatment for, 149–51

triggering in, 12

as two-stage process, 11

N

Nalcrom (disodium cromoglycate), 125, 127

National Institute of Occupational Safety and Health (NIOSH), 104–5

Naturopathy, 108, 109

New Hampshire, indoor air quality legislation in, 102

New Jersey, indoor air quality regulations in, 103

New York, Right to Know Law in, 103–4

Newsprint, sensitivity to, 166

Niagara's Love Canal, 24

Nitrates, 23

Nonbiodegradable detergents, 175

Nonsteroidal anti-inflammatory drugs, 126

Nontoxic cleaning agents, 174

Nutrition. *See* Diet

O

Oasis, setting up personal, 163–67

Occupational Safety and Health Administration (OSHA), 104–5

Omeprazole (Losec), 126

Organochlorine (halogenated) compounds, 185

Oven cleaners, 175

Oxidation, 17

Ozone, 24

Ozone therapy, 109, 110

P

Pea-carrot mixture, 139

Permissible exposure levels (PELs) for toxic chemicals, 83, 104–5

Personal hygiene, temporary changes in, and enzyme potentiated desensitization, 127–28

Pesticides, 23, 184–86

Petroleum products, 185

Pets, 169–70

Phagocytes, 146

Phenol, 181

Phosophoric acids, 176

Phthalates, 27

Pigmentation after cup treatment, 146

Pillows, 165

Pollens, 169

Pollution and multiple chemical sensitivity, 21–27

Polychlorinated biphenyls, 23

Polyunsaturated oils, 153

Polyurethane foam insulation, 183

Potato in enzyme potentiated desensitization diet, 139

Pregnancy and enzyme potentiated desensitization, 123

Product safety sheets, 91–92

Progesterone, 126

Protein, 152, 155

R

Radioacative fallout, 52

Randolph, Theron G., 53–54

Rapp, Doris, 55

Rea, William, 54–55

Reasonable accommodations
making for chemically sensitive employees, 84–85
right to ask for, 100–105

Reduction, 17

Repellents, 169

Resources, 187–220

Reverse osmosis system, 162

Rhubarb, 132

Risks for multiple chemical sensitivity, 41–43

Rotary diet, 156–57
alternative foods for, 159–61
four days of, 157–59
principles of, 157

Rotation diet, 144